GOD BLESS THE NHS

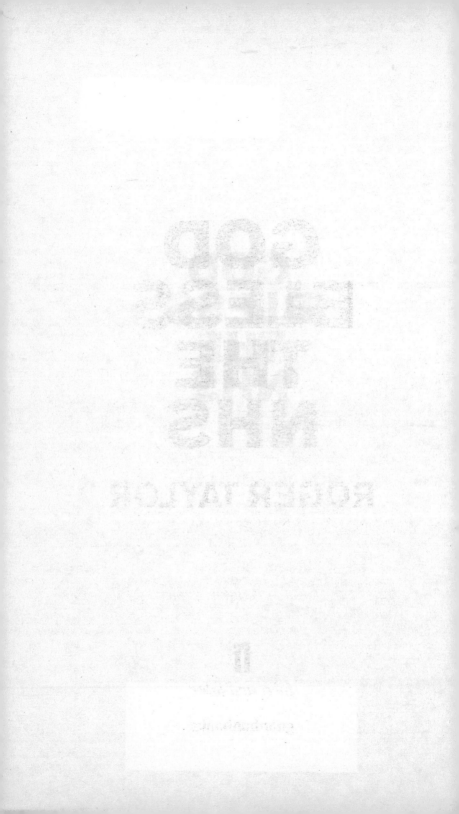

GOD BLESS THE NHS

ROGER TAYLOR

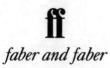

faber and faber

guardianbooks

For Angela Stubbs

First published in 2013
by Faber and Faber Limited
Bloomsbury House
74–77 Great Russell Street
London WC1B 3DA

Published with Guardian Books
Guardian Books is an imprint of Guardian Newspapers Ltd

Text design and typesetting by seagulls.net

Printed and bound in Great Britain by
CPI Group (UK) Ltd, Croydon CR0 4YY

A CIP record for this book is available from the British Library

ISBN 978-0-571-30364-9

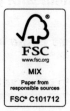

FSC
www.fsc.org
MIX
Paper from
responsible sources
FSC® C101712

2 4 6 8 10 9 7 5 3 1

CONTENTS

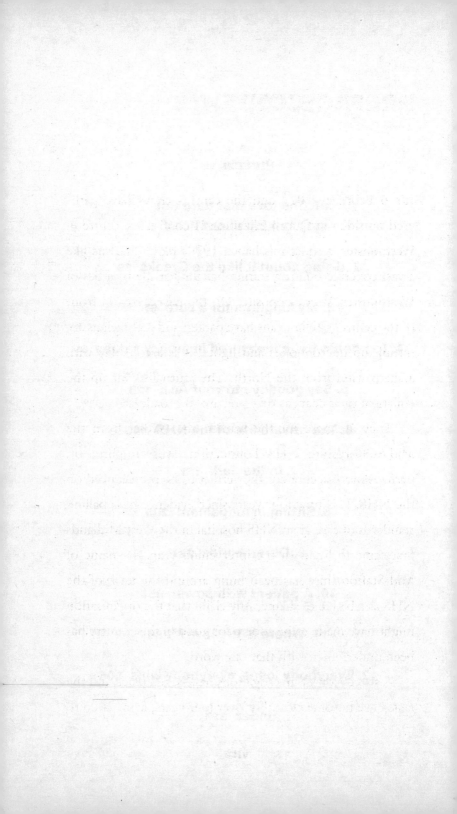

PREFACE

It's 6 February 2013 and the camera crews have gathered outside the Queen Elizabeth II conference centre in Westminster, a squat misshapen 1970s block that sits like a vast concrete bullfrog staring balefully at the beauties of Westminster Abbey opposite. On the paved area in front of the centre, satellite vans have parked and technicians are setting up microphones and lights. It is a cold day with a sharp wind from the North. The journalists lift up the collars of their coats as they prepare to broadcast.

They are here for the verdict, the verdict from the Mid-Staffordshire NHS Foundation Trust inquiry; or, perhaps more accurately, the verdict to be pronounced on the NHS. It is now four years since evidence of appalling standards of care at an NHS hospital in the West Midlands first came to light. In the intervening years the name of Mid-Staffordshire has been hung around the neck of the NHS as a badge of shame. Any claim that the organisation might have made to be a force for good in the country has been undermined with that one word.

A succession of investigations have taken place and the facts have become clear. For over four years, from 2005 to

2009, standards of care in parts of the hospital collapsed. In the emergency department at Stafford Hospital and, most notably, in wards 10 and 11, the lives of patients were turned into a living hell. They were denied vital medical treatments, they were ignored, they were humiliated and left in pain and discomfort. Many spent days and nights on these wards in fear for their safety and scared to complain. For a significant number this was their last experience before they died unnecessarily through lack of decent medical care.

That much is clear. But one question that remains to be answered: who is to blame? Because this is about more than the events that took place in the hospital. This is about the fact that, at various times, there were people at every level of the NHS who had been in a position to spot the problems. There were many who had both the responsibility and the opportunity to intervene. And yet nothing had been done. No one had acted. Guilt by association tainted every part of the NHS.

A lawyer, Robert Francis QC, was appointed to find out what happened. He was asked, in particular, to uncover "why problems at the trust were not identified sooner". Or in other words – who was responsible, who should have done something? The list of suspects was long. The nurses and doctors treating the patients, the board of the hospital, the GPs who referred their patients, the local NHS commissioning organisations, the regional health authorities, the managers in the Department of Health, the regulators and, ultimately, the politicians in Westminster. All of them had some connection to the scene of the crime. But who was guilty?

As the time of the announcement approached the crowd gathered. People arrived who had suffered at the hospital, along with families of people who died there. Many of them had campaigned for years to demand some form of justice. Julie Bailey, whose mother died in Stafford Hospital and who founded the campaign to "Cure the NHS", was there along with many who had given evidence to Robert Francis.

People from the NHS also arrived, heads down, waiting to hear the worst.

When the verdict came there was not so much a gasp as a frown. When all the evidence had been sifted; after the lawyers had carefully judged the behaviour of the politicians, the bureaucrats, the doctors and the nurses; after their claims and counter-claims were weighed and the legal issues considered – it turned out none of them were to blame. It turned out that, all along, lurking in the background like the butler, it was the "culture" that had committed the crime.

The victims and their families were not happy. The culture of the NHS is not something that can apologise and try to atone. The culture of the NHS cannot be punished for its misdeeds. They wanted to see someone held to account. They wanted to know that they were not the only ones to suffer through this disaster. More than anything they wanted to see the chief executive of the NHS forced out of his job.

Jeremy Hunt, the secretary of state for health, had no desire to see his chief executive leave and stood by him. But he too felt something was a bit awry with the verdict. Surely someone, somewhere must be able to carry some of the blame. He suggested that it was now for the police to start investigating the potential criminal liability of those involved in the care of patients.

But the verdict was clear. It was, Robert Francis announced, not possible to castigate "failings on the part of one or even a group of individuals". There was no point in looking for "scapegoats". The guilty party was the "culture of the NHS". It was the culture that had ignored "the priority that should have been given to the protection of patients". It was the culture that "too often did not consider properly the impact on patients of actions being taken".

For the NHS itself the verdict was rather reassuring. Having to atone by trying to change culture is a punishment it can willingly accept. That the NHS needs to change its culture is an accepted mantra among anyone at a senior level inside the organisation. Our health service is replete with experts and project teams working on culture-change initiatives.

While it is easy to understand why many were disappointed by this judgment, there is something that is obviously correct about it. The problems at Mid-Staffordshire reflect faults with the way in which the whole system operates. You could sack whole armies of NHS employees and watch in horror as they were simply replaced by more of the same.

It is right to blame the "culture of the NHS". The challenge is changing it. For over 30 years now professional associations, patient groups and politicians have called for changes in the culture of our healthcare system. Successive governments have produced entire libraries' worth of policies and proposals designed to achieve it. But the problems persist.

The most recent attempt at change was the Coalition government's Health and Social Care Act. Its stated aim was to make the health service more responsive to the needs of patients – exactly what Robert Francis called for.

But its proposed solutions have attracted little support from the public and outright hostility among professionals, prompting doctors to strike.

Will the 290 recommendations from the Mid-Staffordshire inquiry make any difference? Much of what the report proposes is troublingly familiar. It calls for clear standards of care and greater transparency. But then so did the last public inquiry into hospital care. That one took place more than 10 years ago, after it was discovered that surgeons in Bristol had been performing operations on infants which they lacked the skills to do successfully. It too called for clearer standards and greater transparency. Ten years later, here we are again.

It is enough to make the man and woman in the Clapham GP's waiting room despair. How is it possible to have a health system which allows standards of care to persist that all agree are unacceptable but which no one seems capable of stopping? How can the NHS happily accept that it needs to change its ways and yet somehow never manages to fix the problem?

The aim of this book is to provide an overview of the various causes that underlie this paralysis. It matters not just because it led to the tragedies that occurred in Stafford. It matters because it threatens the survival of the NHS.

The culture of the NHS is not a monolithic set of beliefs. It is a culture that has grown out of the conflicting interests and attitudes of the many different groups that form our health services. And that includes more than just politicians, managers and medical professionals. It includes all the rest of us too. The NHS is a national institution in which we all play a part, as citizens, patients, voters and carers, even if we are not one of the million people employed by it.

I have attempted to review the main areas of greatest controversy as these best illustrate the difficulties. For example, there is the conflict between the private and public sector that has flared up in the light of plans to privatise more NHS services. Then there are the battles between the NHS and local communities over efforts to reorganise local services. And in the background, behind all of this, there is the constant struggle between doctors and managers over who is in charge.

Of all the culture wars in the NHS, the rift between those who are responsible for the money and those who are responsible for looking after patients is perhaps the most fundamental. Over 35 years ago, Robert Alford, a US sociologist, first identified this as the fundamental conflict in modern healthcare. He also observed that in the often vicious scrapping between these parties, the patient was largely powerless. Like the children of squabbling parents, we sit in the back seat of the car, stare out of the window and hope that the bickering will stop.

It is sometimes argued that the problems of poor care and financial problems are unrelated. After all, treating the frail and the sick with respect is surely an issue that transcends finance. But if you need an example of how these issues cannot be separated, look no further than Mid-Staffordshire. While it is true that many instances of poor care were down to people simply failing to act as they should, it is also true that the problems were precipitated by cuts in staff numbers implemented by the board of a hospital that was struggling to make ends meet financially.

Over the coming years the single biggest influence on the way the NHS changes will be the increasingly stringent financial pressures. If we apply that to a culture which responds by letting standards collapse, we are all in for a very rough ride.

This book is about the culture of the NHS in its broadest sense. It is as much about the culture and attitudes of those receiving healthcare as those providing it. We are all part of the NHS. To the extent that there are cultural problems, it is as much about our attitudes to how we want to be looked after as it is about the attitudes of those who are paid to care for us.

We have much to gain from trying to change the culture of the NHS. Robert Francis is right when he says it is putting patients' lives at risk. Equally, it is putting the future of our health service at risk. Fixing the culture is in all of our interests. But it is also something that can only be achieved with the involvement of all of us.

My connection with the NHS is an odd one and probably needs explaining. I am not a doctor. I have never been employed by the NHS. I have never even been sufficiently sick to be a long-term patient of the health service. I am by background a journalist who began his career working for Which? magazine, trying to identify dodgy insurance salesmen. My involvement with health services began 12 years ago. I had been reporting for the Financial Times in San Francisco. It was during the early period of the growth of the internet and I was fascinated by the way that technology was making it possible to use information in new ways.

In 1999, my father died. My mother, living back in Kent, was suffering from worsening Parkinson's disease. My wife was about to give birth to our second child. It seemed like the moment to move back to England. So we came home and I started to look for something new to do.

It was then that Tim Kelsey, who was news editor at the Sunday Times, called me with what seemed at the time a simple plan – to set up a company that would tell people which hospitals and which doctors were good and which were not. It seemed worthwhile. It felt like something I could help make to happen. So I said yes.

We established ourselves in an office in Old Street in 2000 and very quickly discovered just how far from simple this plan was going to be. The technical challenges of assessing quality in healthcare were significant. But the political and cultural challenge was much bigger. I was astonished to find that, in the eyes of many people involved in the NHS, this was not regarded as a worthwhile exercise at all. Many regarded it as actively hostile.

Not everyone felt this way. In particular a number of doctors and the more politically astute in the NHS felt that what we were doing was needed. Crucially, one GP in particular felt very differently – Professor Sir Brian Jarman, who as well as practising as a doctor in London, was a statistician at Imperial College. He was deeply troubled at what his analysis of hospital mortality rates seemed to show in terms of the standards of care in some parts of the NHS. It was these figures which, some years later, were to trigger the investigations into Mid-Staffordshire NHS Foundation Trust.

In 2001, the first Dr Foster Hospital Guide was published, including Professor Jarman's analysis of mortality rates. It was treated with suspicion and anger through much of the health service. As a journalist I had written about and commented on many walks of life. But I had never encountered any area of activity where criticism prompted such indignant fury. It was my first encounter with some of the less attractive aspects of NHS culture.

Since then, Dr Foster has found a way to coexist with the NHS and the NHS has become more open than it was. But change has been slow and the culture of the NHS remains one that is inward-looking, one that is mistrustful of outsiders and one that is often too quick to accept good intentions as an excuse for poor results.

There is a phrase used in the health service, the "NHS family". It refers to all the organisations and individuals that are seen to share the values and objectives of the NHS. It is a pretty loose confederation but those who are part of the family know who they are. Dr Foster is now half-owned by the NHS and has become part of the family, albeit a rather distant relation. So the perspective I bring is neither quite the view of an insider nor the view of an outsider. I have spent most of the past decade talking to doctors and NHS managers about how they can better understand information about the standards of care they are providing, and to patients and patient groups about how they understand these issues.

My views are informed by these conversations and by my own experiences but I should stress that the opinions expressed in this book are mine and do not reflect the views of either Dr Foster or anyone who is, or has been, involved in the organisation. There are a great many people I would like to thank for their wise advice on this book but I will not list them, not least as some of them were charmingly direct about the degree to which they disagreed with the way I have presented some of the more contentious debates.

Most of the issues discussed in this book are covered much more authoritatively by others. In particular, I would point anyone interested in reading further to the following: for an account of the politics behind the Health and Social Care Act, Never Again, by Nick Timmins, published by the Institute of Government; on the implications of the growing complexity of healthcare and the potential for technological advance in medicine, Chaos and Organization in Health Care, by Tom Lee and James Mongan; for an assessment of the economic challenges facing the NHS, Securing Our Future Health: Taking the Long-term View, by Derek Wanless, along with the updates to that report; on the difficulties of making healthcare reliable, Patient Safety, by Charles Vincent; and, on the need for patients to be given greater control over their healthcare, Towards the Emancipation of Patients, by Charlotte Williamson.

CHAPTER 1

The love that dare not stop talking about itself

The American author AJ Jacobs coined a term for it: auto-schadenfreude – the joy we take in our own misfortune. It is something the British do well. At times it becomes an urgent and all-consuming exercise. Such was the mood of the population of Britain as the London 2012 Olympics approached and we contemplated with grim delight how badly the opening ceremony would suck. We confidently expected a national humiliation.

The problem was Beijing. There has been an arms race in Olympic opening ceremonies over recent decades with each host nation expected to top whatever has come before. Our misfortune was to come four years after China, earth's most populous nation and its second biggest economy, threw everything it had into creating an opening ceremony to make the jaw of the world drop.

It succeeded. Some of what took place in the Bird's Nest stadium was down to electronic trickery, but that did not stop the sense of awe as a giant luminous scroll unfurled across the floor of arena. Dancers moved across it with brush-like movements, causing calligraphy to appear. Then hundreds more dancers entered, moving with perfect synchronicity. As they formed the shapes of printing machines and Chinese characters, it was hard to believe that this really was a team of dancers and not a machine

Britain resigned itself to the idea that nothing we did could match it. We grumbled that anyone can put on a decent show given a workforce of more than a billion with no democratic rights. But we feared that our own effort would display such shaming amateurishness that the only possible response would be to laugh about it.

It has become customary for the host nation to use the opening ceremony to give an account of its history and place in the world. In Athens in 2004, moving tableaux told us about ancient Greece's contribution to the development of theatre, philosophy, maths and art. The Chinese used their magic scroll to remind us that they were the font of much of modern civilisation. Writing with ink, paper-making and printing are all things that first happened in China. London decided to stick with the format. We would tell our island story with three hours of music, dance and visual effects.

The ceremony began with the inside of the stadium converted into a slice of idealised British countryside.

Villagers played cricket and football. Shakespeare was read. Elgar played. Then huge chimneys erupted from the ground as Britain's role leading the Industrial Revolution was re-enacted. Huge Olympic rings were forged from rivers of molten iron and then lifted high above the stadium.

The country rocked back on its heels and enjoyed the unexpected sensation of having its cynicism blown away. This was impressive. It was spectacular, it was exciting and it was about us. Cricket, Shakespeare, the industrial revolution – these things were British, they were great. They were what we had brought to the world.

Then it all went a bit peculiar. From all sides of the stadium came doctors and nurses pushing children in hospital beds. The logo of Great Ormond Street Hospital appeared. Next, the centre of the stadium was filled with three letters in white lights. NHS. Danny Boyle, the creator of the opening ceremony, had decided to use the occasion to tell the world how proud we were of our health service.

To anyone born and brought up in Britain it seemed natural. From the hotel bar in Turkey, where I watched the ceremony, it seemed decidedly odd. The commentators offered no guidance as foreign audiences struggled to make sense of things. Why are they telling us about their hospitals? Will the Rio Olympics in four years' time include a ballet on the Brazilian state pension scheme?

Why did the Chinese not tell us more about their national rail network?

The choreographed nurses segued into a section on children's literature. The link was the fact that the royalties from JM Barrie's Peter Pan were donated to Great Ormond Street Hospital for Children. Wicked characters, including the child snatcher from Chitty Chitty Bang Bang and orcs from the Hobbit, began to menace the kids, who leapt up and down on their beds in fear. Rescue came in the form of a squadron of Mary Poppinses, parachuting from above on umbrellas.

Children's literature is another area where Britain has done much that resonates around the world from Robert Louis Stevenson to JK Rowling. But healthcare? What were we saying about healthcare? Watching the spectacle of NHS patients being rescued by fictional nannies seemed to say more about our national psyche than was perhaps intended.

Commentators were divided. Some professed utter bewilderment – particularly those in the US. Most were confused but charmed. Ai Weiwei the Chinese dissident artist who designed the Bird's Nest stadium, was kind, writing in the Observer newspaper: "It was very, very well done. This was about Great Britain. It didn't pretend it was trying to have global appeal."

It is a generous sentiment. But he underestimates how important we think we are. He does not appreciate the degree to which the British do believe the NHS is an organisation of global significance.

The show was filled with things that we wanted the world to know were ours – James Bond, the monarchy, British pop music. There was even a rather toe-curling claim to have played a big part in the development of the internet on the grounds that Tim Berners-Lee, the guy who set up the world wide web (while employed in Geneva), happens to be a Brit. Tim was duly displayed sitting at a desk in the middle of a packed Olympic Stadium looking like nothing so much as the re-enactment of an anxiety dream.

One thing came through very clearly. The NHS is part of our national story. It is part of our national myth. We think it says something important about who we are.

We love our health service. We love it in a way that has no parallel in other countries. Compared with the rest of the world, few people in Britain call into question the healthcare system. In one 2012 study, only 3 per cent of people felt the system needed to be overhauled. The next most satisfied country has more than twice as many people questioning their arrangements. It compares with a rate of about 10 per cent across Europe and 25 per cent in the US.

The social consensus is so strong around the NHS that dissenting voices sound jarring. When a Conservative member of the European Parliament, Daniel Hannan, described the NHS as a "mistake" on US TV, there was genuine shock and surprise back home. David Cameron described his opinion as "eccentric". He was right. People in Britain do not hold views like that.

It is not unusual to hear people protest that they "will not hear a word said against" the NHS. Criticism can quickly become blasphemy. And the praise at times becomes daft. Take this example from the Times,* in which Caitlin Moran, in a review of a TV programme about the NHS wrote: "Oh, the fabulous luxury of the NHS: the only profligacy that isn't profligacy at all – but some rare blend of care, civilisation and sanity that still feels like one of the great wonders of the world. For all the good it has done, has humanity ever topped its brilliance – even in the Great Pyramid or Rhapsody in Blue?" She goes on to say how, in other countries, people would wake in their hospital beds and be presented with the bill. But here, with the NHS, you wake surrounded by relieved and grateful loved ones.

She sums up how many people in Britain feel. We believe that the NHS is a remarkable and unusual

---

* Times, Review, It's the best time to accidently cut your own leg off, 19 May 2012.

arrangement. We believe that is it different and ahead of what goes on in other countries. Many people believe that the very idea of universal healthcare – making sure everyone can access healthcare when they need it regardless of wealth – is an idea invented in Britain and uniquely realised in Britain. None of this is true. But it but it leads us to hold the institution of the NHS in a peculiar reverence.

When Tory peer Nigel Lawson described the NHS as our only national religion, he was not being flippant. Nothing unites us so much as our health service. No other country holds its healthcare system in such pious regard. To Britons it is obvious why the NHS featured so prominently in the Olympic ceremony.

This attitude to our health service raises something of a mystery – a mystery about our politics and our politicians, a puzzle that to many people can only be explained by the existence of secret conspiracies and hidden agendas.

The mystery is this: why on earth, when everybody is so delighted with the NHS, do politicians endlessly embark on trying to change it? Why do successive governments insisting on trying to redesign the system? Why are we endlessly shutting down one set of NHS organisations and replacing them with a new set?

To have given a proper account of the NHS, the Olympic opening ceremony should really have included a short mime of NHS managers being handed redundancy notices.

In the first half of the of the NHS's 60-year existence it underwent only one major reorganisation. In 1974, the Conservative government put each part of the country under the management of an area health authority. In the next two decades it underwent two re-organisations – in 1982 and 1991, when the "internal market" was introduced. This separated the NHS into bodies that "bought" or "commissioned" services on behalf of the public and those that provided them.

Over the next 10 years, under Labour, reorganisations started to come thick and fast with at least four major restructurings in one decade, depending on how you count the endless changes. On the trajectory set by New Labour we were moving rapidly towards a state of permanent revolution with structures dismantled almost the moment they had achieved a stable and routine way of working. A period of stability was called for. Then the Coalition arrived.

There is a common plot device used in alien invasion films. Earth comes under attack from robotic assault craft of such advanced technology that resistance seems futile. Relying on nothing more than ingenuity and guts, humans start to fight back. Victory seems possible. Then the sky darkens. We look up to see the assault craft dwindle into specks as the mother-ship descends, blotting out the sun and raining destruction below.

If Labour's reforms were the alien assault craft, the Coalition's Health and Social Care Bill was the mother-ship. The fight moved to a whole new level.

Every reform of the NHS is met with objections. Doctors and nurses complain and the public shake their heads in despair. The Labour government from 1997 to 2010 enjoyed a degree of public permission to mess around with health because it had successfully argued that we should double the amount of money we paid into it. But for the Coalition no such latitude was given. Indeed, in opposition the Conservatives had promised specifically not to reorganise the NHS, being aware of just how unpopular such a move would be.

So why did they do it? The mystery is deepened by the fact that when the Coalition came to power in 2010, approval for the NHS was stronger than ever. (While *support* for the NHS as an institution is always strong, public *approval* wavers – when waiting lists get too long, for example, or hospitals too filthy.) In government surveys, it was getting positive ratings from 70 per cent of respondents – the highest figure achieved as far as records go back.* Quite

---

* British Social Attitudes survey, 2011. Data goes back 28 years.

likely, this was the highest satisfaction rating that the NHS has ever enjoyed.

For any national institution to command the support of 97 per cent of the population and the approval of more than two-thirds is a remarkable achievement. For an institution that employs over one million people and regularly and directly affects the lives of every citizen in delivering a highly complex service; for an institution that is the subject of continuous political debate and scrutiny by regulators, academics and experts; for an institution that is subject to criticism in the press every day – it is little short of a miracle.

In these circumstances, what could have possessed David Cameron to start taking apart what he rightly dubbed "our most treasured national asset"?

It is not as if there was nothing else to keep him busy. We were in the grip of the most serious economic crisis since the 1930s; unpopular cuts were being pushed through; the government was an untested and potentially fragile coalition with no one party in control of the House of Commons. Surely this was not the time to start messing with the one institution in the country that enjoyed near unanimous support.

It was not ignorance that encouraged Cameron to act. Politicians understand the place of the NHS in people's hearts. They fall over each other protesting their love for it. In the debate over the Coalition's healthcare reforms, Labour leader Ed Miliband ran his campaign under the banner "We love the NHS." Like a creepily possessive boyfriend, David Cameron replied: "It's because I love the NHS so much that I want to change it."

One answer to the mystery is that it is a huge cock-up – that the hurried negotiations after the election to agree a health policy with the Liberal Democrats produced a compromise that no one really agreed with. Or that the bill which resulted was rushed out before anyone outside the Department of Health fully understood the implications of what was being proposed. It was only when the Department of Health advisers came over to No. 10 to properly explain what was being proposed that the penny dropped and Cameron famously exclaimed, "We're fucked."

Cock-up certainly played an important role, as has been described in fascinating detail by Nicholas Timmins in his excellent account of the process by which the 2010 Health and Social Care Bill came into being.* This book is not about that. This book is about why, when confronted with this situation, David Cameron chose to back the healthcare reforms at a very high political cost to himself and his party.

----

* See Nicholas Timmins, Never Again? The Story of the Health and Social Care Act 2012. London: King's Fund, 2012.

It took nearly two years of gruelling hand-to-hand combat to force the Health and Social Care Bill through the Houses of Parliament against widespread public and professional opposition. Those against it included the British Medical Association, the Royal College of General Practitioners, the Royal College of Nurses, the Royal College of Midwives, the Faculty of Public Health and the Patients Association. As the debate raged, doctors went on strike for the first time since 1974. Public satisfaction with what was happening in the NHS plummeted as the bickering intensified.

At the height of the argument, Andrew Lansley, then Secretary of State for Health, found himself being chased down the corridors of the Royal Marsden Hospital by a doctor of 30 years standing who was angrily shouting his opposition to the reforms. Except it was not really opposition but confusion. "Explain to me how this bill is going to make patients better", he yelled, "because no one understands your bill."

It was not a pithy slogan – not compared to the banners being held by the protesters outside the hospital – but very much to the point. What problem, exactly, are the current reforms to the NHS supposed to fix?

Very few people – and certainly not many of the people involved in delivering the health service – have any clear idea why this is happening. The government has failed to provide any coherent account of what it is trying to do and why. It has said it wants to improve the quality of the NHS. But, as we have seen, people were happier than they ever had been with it. There are many aspects of the NHS that could be improved; that has always been the case and will always remain the case. But there was no public outcry demanding improvement. What possible political gain would the government achieve by pushing forward with proposals that were so patently unpopular?

It has said it wants to provide more power to patients and communities. But who are the patients and the communities demanding this power? I am very strong advocate of giving greater power to patients and communities – and in the course of this book I will explain why. But anyone who is an advocate of patient power knows that one of the biggest hurdles to overcome is the deep ambivalence patients feel about being asked to take more control over their healthcare, and more responsibility for it. There are very few votes in promising to give the public more power over the NHS.

So what is really going on? Why do we keep dismantling and rebuilding the NHS? The aim of this book is to unpick exactly how we got into this curious position. I want to uncover the real reasons why, at a time of crisis elsewhere, the government has decided to spend a great deal of money and even larger amounts of political capital fixing perhaps the only thing in Britain that people didn't feel was broken.

To the audience crowded into the Friends House on Euston Road on 23 June 2012, David Cameron's motive is obvious.

Frances O'Grady, General Secretary of the TUC, spells it out: "This is not about quality, this is not about giving power to communities, this is about the nasty rightwing agenda of turning patients into profits."

She may be preaching to the home crowd but she is a fine speaker and knows how to get an audience charged. She knows that the provisions in the NHS Health and Social Care Act to allow the private sector to take over parts of the NHS is the issue that has caused greatest opposition.

I am at Reclaiming Our NHS, a national conference organised by the NHS Support Federation and Keep Our NHS Public, a coalition of different interest groups opposed to the reforms. These are the people most committed to halting the reform programme. Looking round the room, there is a sense of history – a feeling that this could be any radical movement meeting over the last 100 years.

The audience are not afraid to heckle and will on occasions shout out angry challenges to speakers.

There are no suits here, no high fashion. I am reminded of the Labour party meetings I used to attend in the 1980s. Looking round the room, I suspect many of the individuals may have similar memories. Like me, they are mainly grey-haired and middle-aged. An elderly Sikh stands up at one point to ask: "Where are all the young people? We need the support of the youth."

As is traditional at such meetings, there is a pleasing if eccentric sense of chaos and democratic inclusiveness. At one point a GP from south London stands up to read out an email from a group of doctors in Egypt who wish to express their support for the campaign, comparing it to the battles they have had to fight against the recently toppled Mubarak regime.

The contributions from the podium are equally diverse. A woman in pink tights and a yellow head scarf talks about the need for "theatrical events" that will engage the public, such as mock auctions of NHS hospitals. She calls for protests outside Virgin shops because Virgin Care, part of Richard Branson's business empire, is seeking to run community services for the NHS. She wants a sit-in at the offices of Circle, a business which has recently taken over the running of Hinchinbrooke Hospital from the NHS.

O'Grady's speech is full of history. She talks of the NHS as "one of this country's defining achievements ... a socialist achievement ... founded in the aftermath of the second world war in the teeth of opposition from the conservative establishment." At the same time she is trying to be forward-looking. She talks about the need to work with digital activists in the "progressive movement". But the phrase feels wrong. The progressive movement? It sounds antique, pre-war, of a piece with the 1930s architecture of the hall.

She reaches the climax of her speech, raising her voice above the cheers and clapping. The NHS "is a socialist achievement based on collective action. It is about the strong helping the weak and everyone having access to care. So it is urgent that we defend the public ethos that lies at the heart of the NHS. The overwhelming majority of NHS professionals are on our side and the majority of the British people are on our side." The audience stand and applaud.

The history of the NHS, the way it came into being, is a big part of our national myth. It was done at a stroke with a single act by a reforming government elected in the aftermath of the second world war. It was an act of remarkable political bravery and vision which set Britain apart from its fellow nations.

Before 1948, the liberal reforms of 1911 had ensured access to healthcare for workers but coverage was neither universal (families and those out of work were often not covered) nor comprehensive (the insurance did not guarantee to meet all healthcare needs). There were community hospitals, run by local authorities, that were available to ratepayers, but not to non-ratepayers. In 1948, with the introduction of the NHS, Aneurin Bevan created a system that provided comprehensive healthcare for all while at the same time taking almost every hospital in the country into national ownership and making the majority of nurses and hospital doctors employees of the state.

The scope of the new system made the Britain an example that other countries looked up to. O'Grady is right to describe it as one of the country's defining achievements. It is something we can be proud of.

But that is history and history happened a long time ago. The creation of the NHS was a great day for our nation. But then so was winning the Battle of Trafalgar. The one says as much about the state of our health services today as the other says about the state of the British navy.

Because the NHS was unusual when it was created, there is a tendency among some in Britain to think that it must still be very unusual today. In particular, there is at times the idea – even among very senior politicians –

that universal healthcare, the provision of healthcare to all, when they need it, regardless of their ability to pay, is something that other countries do not do.

The Germans actually got there first. Otto von Bismarck was the first politician – back in 1883 – to introduce legislation to ensure everyone could see a doctor when they needed to, regardless of whether they had the money to pay. The Germans, like many other countries, use a compulsory insurance system rather than tax to fund care but it achieves similar results. Everyone must be insured and those who can't afford it are paid for by the government.

Today, outside the US, virtually every developed country provides universal comprehensive healthcare. The French are just as proud as the British about the fact that, whoever you are, in France, if you need medical attention you will get it. The Germans do not regard their citizens as any less well cared-for than the British. The Dutch, the Danes, the Swedes, Norwegians and the Finns can say with pride that their commitment to equality in healthcare is second to none.

Some of these systems are paid for out of taxation. Some are paid for through compulsory insurance. In some of these systems, the state is the main provider of care, as in the UK. In others, private and voluntary organisations provide the services. But the objective is the same – to ensure that all citizens can be sure to get the care they need, when they need it.

There are differences between national systems. An important measure of a universal healthcare system is how much people pay for healthcare out of their own pocket. This can either be in the form of "co-payments", where the patient is required to make a contribution to the care guaranteed by the state; or in the form of "top-up payments", where the patient chooses to pay for additional services over and above the care usually provided.

The UK scores well on this measure. There are almost no co-payments required from NHS patients. The only example is the £7.65 fee for prescriptions. Most countries – whether tax-funded or insurance-funded – require most patients to pay something towards the costs of seeing a doctor or receiving care. As a result, the UK has very few people who complain of not being able to get healthcare because of financial worries.

The UK also has relatively low levels of top-up payment. Few people in the UK choose to pay for healthcare over and above that provided by the state. Total private expenditure in the UK is lower than in most EU countries. Only Denmark and the Netherlands have lower rates.*

---

* OECD 2011–12 Factbook. Private expenditure on healthcare as per cent of total healthcare spending 2009.

So on this basis the UK can claim to have one of the more egalitarian health systems in the world. However, these are not the only measures of a health system. Another issue is the extent of the service provided. Just how comprehensive is comprehensive? Some European systems cover a much wider range of activities than the UK – for example, they may include long-term nursing care, dental care and opticians' services – aspects of which are not part of the free NHS cover in England.

The quality and availability of services also matter. The UK has fewer doctors per head and fewer intensive care beds than most European countries. Less provision of healthcare is likely to affect the poor far more than the rich since the poor suffer higher rates of ill-health. In Germany, there is much more private spending on healthcare than in the UK. But the level of public spending per head on healthcare is also higher than in the UK.

So while the NHS can claim to be a good example of universal comprehensive healthcare, it does not obviously outshine other European systems. Certainly, the idea that our approach to healthcare is fundamentally different from what goes on elsewhere in the world is wrong.

Our national attitude to the NHS is not explained by anything particularly striking about the NHS itself. Our healthcare arrangements are neither particularly brilliant, nor unusually bad. In international comparisons, the NHS is somewhere in the middle of the league tables – usually closer to the top than the bottom.* We tend to do well in terms of satisfaction with the service and poorly in terms of health outcomes and in terms of treating people with respect. But whatever aspect we are looking at, like most health systems, we do very well on some measures, but very poorly on others.

When Caitlin Moran gushes that the NHS is one of humanity's great achievements, she is mixing up a lot of things. Much of her admiration comes from her astonishment at the ability of doctors to save people's lives. She is right to be astonished – this does indeed rank among the greatest achievements of humanity. But modern medicine and the NHS are not the same thing.

Modern medicine deserves hyperbolic descriptions. Highly skilled people working in high-pressure environments using some of the most remarkable technology ever developed to overcome what, at times, seem insurmountable odds to restore people to health is awe-inspiring. But the NHS is not a particularly awe-inspiring example of modern medicine. It has some shining examples of

---

* See for example D Ingleby et al., How the NHS measures up to other health systems. BMJ, 2012: 344. doi: 10.1136/bmj.e1079

world-class brilliance, but it also has some distinctly less impressive examples of poor practice.

Our relationship with the NHS is better explained by the way it came into existence. Because the NHS was created as a single national entity, we have a single national brand that encompasses almost every aspect of the healthcare we receive. The letters NHS represent the whole package: they stand for social equality and universal healthcare; they stand for the doctors and the nurses who treat us or our relatives and to whom we are grateful; they stand for the miracles performed daily by modern medicine; they stand for the financial systems that make sure we don't have to worry about paying.

It is hard for people in other countries to feel such a strong attachment to their national healthcare system because there is often no obvious brand to which sentiments can attach. It is hard to imagine how people could feel a similar sense of loyalty to their health insurance policy or the particular hospital in their town.

When it comes to the people who care for us, there is a basic human need to give them our trust and respect. When we are saved from danger, regardless of whether this has been done well or poorly, it is impossible not to feel a deep sense of gratitude. The UK is unusual in that, to a large degree, the emotions that attach to the people and the particular institutions that look after us also attach to our national system of healthcare delivery.

This can result in confusion. When people criticise the NHS, it can seem as if they are denigrating the heroic individual who saved your mother's life or the value of modern medicine. This can undermine our ability to talk sensibly about health.

At times, praise of the NHS replaces patriotism as the last resort of scoundrels. British politicians no longer wrap themselves in the flag, they wrap themselves in the blue and white of the NHS logo. When a politician says he loves the NHS, it is time to start asking some difficult questions.

When David Cameron says he loves the NHS what exactly is he referring to? Is it the nurses and doctors he has come into contact with? Or does he mean the institutions and organisations within which so many NHS employees work? Presumably not the latter, since his government has abolished so many of them.

Take Mr Cameron's declaration of love given in a speech at Ealing Hospital in May 2011, when he announced he would be proceeding with the reforms: "We love the NHS because it's there when the people we love fall ill. Because it's there all the time. Because whoever you are, wherever you are from, however much money you have got in the bank, there's somewhere to go to get looked after. And because that says amazing things about our country. That's why we love the NHS."

Note the claim that having a system of universal healthcare says amazing things about our country. It does not. Well, no more than the amazing things the French healthcare system says about the French and the German healthcare system says about the Germans. And yet we still like to kid ourselves about this. Also, see how the use of the term "NHS" makes it possible to talk nonsense without anyone really noticing. Replace "NHS" in the sentences above with any specific part of the NHS and the absurdity of it becomes clear. We love Dorchester Hospital because it is there all the time?

Ed Miliband is equally a beneficiary of this vagueness. When he says he loves the NHS is he saying he loves universal healthcare? Or does he means he loves state ownership of health services? Or perhaps he is happiest if the distinction gets lost in the heat of the debate. One thing he does not mean is that the NHS is just fine the way it is. Like David Cameron, he loves the NHS so much that he knows he needs to change it, even if that means "difficult and sometimes unpopular choices".[*]

---

[*]   Ed Miliband, The future of the NHS. Speech to the RSA, 4 April 2011. For transcript see: "To protect the NHS is to change it" at www. newstatesman.com/uk-politics/2011/04/nhs-patients-future-change

Everyone loves the NHS the same way everyone loves a newborn baby. Not to love the NHS would be inhuman. By the same token, to express love for the NHS is expected, indeed required, but tells you almost nothing about what that person actually thinks.

Back in Friends House, Dr Jacky Davis is next up on the podium. She is a consultant radiologist at the Whittington Hospital in North London and co-chair of the NHS Consultants' Association. She has a track record of organising effective opposition to changes to the NHS. In 2004, she attacked the Labour government's plans to allow patients to choose where they were treated. She called it a "smokescreen for the government's intention to privatise the NHS". In 2010, she helped lead a march of 5,000 Camden residents against plans to close the accident and emergency department of her hospital. To date, the A&E remains open.

She lacks the oratory of O'Grady, but she knows the arguments in detail and begins to point out flaws in the Health and Social Care Act, clause by clause. The forced passage of the act was, she says, "a low point for democracy in this country". It is "a bottle of snake oil" that will not give power to patients but will lead to GPs having to answer to commissioning groups run by private companies. It will mean patients being refused treatments and care becoming confused with "a ragbag of competing companies and the NHS reduced to a logo – patients won't even know who is providing their care".

"This is a purely ideological attack on the NHS," she says. The government are using the financial crisis to attack public services and, in particular, the NHS because it is so successful. "A successful public service is an anathema to these free-marketeers."

She starts to pick off the enemy one by one: Care UK, a private company running a number of treatment centres for NHS patients which has made significant donations to Andrew Lansley's campaign funds; and Virgin Care, which has just won the contract to manage the formerly NHS-run community health services in Surrey, and whose commercial director has just been invited by Andrew Lansley to sit on the committee reviewing the NHS Constitution.

It is clear what is happening – it is a plot, a conspiracy in which capitalist profit-making organisations have financed politicians who have then imposed changes on the NHS against the will of the people. The fat contracts they get doing NHS work will fill their coffers and enable them to buy up even more politicians and reward their loyal servants with well-paid jobs after they have left office. The only rational response is revolution.

It is rare to see middle-aged NHS consultants openly calling for rebellion, but these are unusual times. Davis says the time has come to refuse to co-operate. She calls for occupations and a boycott of the private sector. She quotes Gandhi. "When the government turns against the people, rebellion is a responsibility."

It is easy to see why people come to the view that privatisation of the NHS is part of an anti-democratic conspiracy by shady capitalist forces. There is a certain logic to it. When O'Grady says the majority of healthcare professionals and the majority of the public are against these reforms, the opinion polls back her up.[*] And yet the politicians persist. If a government is trying to push something through against the will of the people they must be in hock to some interest group.

The inability of politicians to be open does not help. The Tories decided not to talk about their health policy in the run up to the 2010 election on the grounds that people found the details of NHS organisation tedious. Mr Lansley had in fact been very clear about his plans in a large number of public statements prior to the election campaign. But during the campaign nothing was said apart from the promise not to carry out another "top-down reorganisation".

---

[*]   For example, the Department of Health's own Public Perceptions of the NHS and Social Care Survey from Ipsos/Mori.

The excuse put forward when the Coalition unveiled their plans – that the reforms were "bottom-up" not "top-down" – was straight out of the playground: "I didn't hit him, Sir, he pushed his face on my hand".

Then there is the way the different policies interact with each other. The government is currently holding down the level of NHS funding below the level needed to meet increasing demand. This is being done, it says, because of the need to reduce the high levels of government debt following the 2008 financial crisis. The government says the only option is for the NHS to become more efficient.

At the same time the government is inviting private companies to start providing more NHS services *and* they are freeing up NHS hospitals to start offering more private care.

To the conspiracy theorists, the intention is obvious. The NHS, which is already more efficient than many other health services, will be unable to cope with the financial pressure and services will be withdrawn. At the same time, the organisations providing care – both NHS and private – will be able to offer privately funded services to replace them. Quietly, without anyone noticing, the NHS will be dismantled.

Guardian journalist Polly Toynbee, speaking as part of a panel at the end of the day in Friends House, hints at the hidden agenda. The Health and Social Care Act, she says, is the one that "really levers open what this government is all about".

But accusations of bad faith can be applied to all sides in this debate. Many in the room are aware of the tension. It is there when one speaker from the floor complains about how their movement is portrayed in the media as being "vested interests" rather than a real movement of communities. This only highlights the fact that the speakers are almost all union representatives or work in the health and social care services. It is they who stand to lose most if private organisations start to compete.

Opponents of the reforms may question politicians' motivation. But they know they face an equally big challenge persuading people that their vision is driven by more than self-interest. After all, what sort of political manifesto would unite the diverse constituencies gathered together on the Euston Road. It is hard to believe that the Communist Party of Great Britain, Unison, the NHS Consultants' Association and the Royal College of General Practitioners have anything in common apart from an alliance of convenience.

The claims of hidden agendas and conspiracies are born of understandable frustration – frustration that, despite widespread public opposition to privatisation and

NHS reform, every government insists on continuing the process. Politicians may, in opposition, express doubts about their rivals' proposals. But once in power they invariably do the same thing. Like most conspiracy theories, this one founders on the astonishingly wide number of people who would need to be involved in it for the theory to stand up – from Gordon Brown and the current chief executive of the NHS, David Nicholson (a former communist) to Nick Clegg and David Cameron.

This is the real problem that opponents of the reforms face – they have few real friends in power. One of the biggest cheers of the day goes to a young woman who goes up to the podium and says: "We have been wrong to rely on the Labour party … The Labour party sold out to Milton Friedman many years ago … It is now dedicated to privatisation and the free market." But the audience becomes more unsettled as she follows her argument to its logical conclusion. The crisis, she says, is a crisis in the representation of the people. "We need a new party and we need to build it," she says. She is right. They do need a new party. But what happened with all the old ones? Why did they all abandon them?

Many journalists and politicians like to characterise the fight over the NHS Health and Social Care Act as a struggle between right and left, between the values of Socialism and the values of Conservatism. This is a fiction that serves to make politicians look more heroic.

The reality is rather different. If you were to take a group of policy advisers working in the Labour party or the Conservative party and ask them to set out the issues facing the NHS, you would find that the vast majority agree on pretty well all the major points. There is no major ideological divide over the future of the NHS. If anything, there is a rather alarming degree of consensus across the political spectrum among anyone within sniffing distance of power. Both sides support allowing the private sector to provide NHS services, both sides support keeping services free at the point of delivery, both sides support retaining a tax-funded system of finance, both sides support greater clinician involvement in spending decisions, both sides support more choice and competition, both sides recognise the need for greater integration.

When the Conservatives first laid out their plans in 2006, they were widely seen as nothing more than a continuation of the policies being pursued by Tony Blair.* But this extraordinary level of agreement does not stop parliament, like a candy floss machine, whipping up great clouds

---

* See Timmins, Never Again, for a more complete account.

of important-sounding debate out of issues of almost no consequence.

Take the strenuous argument in the Lords about the role of the Health Secretary in the running of the NHS. Across the political spectrum there has been recognition for some time that political interference in the NHS can be a problem. If a way could be found to put some distance between day-to-day NHS decisions and politics it might improve the quality of the decisions. There has been, quite rightly, some scepticism that this is possible since, whatever structures are in place, the public are likely to continue to hold the government electorally responsible for the NHS and politicians are likely to act accordingly. But it is worth trying. Gordon Brown in 2006 suggested in an interview that an independent board to run the NHS might be a good idea. When the Conservatives announced it as their policy, Rosie Winterton, a Labour health minister, said it was an idea worth looking at.

Fast-forward five years to the publication of the Health and Social Care Bill. Right at the top is a clause which limits the secretary of state's responsibility for delivering the health service and moves it to a new independent commissioning board. This is one of the flashpoints for opposition to the bill. Furious speeches complain that the government would no longer be obliged to provide comprehensive healthcare and that the future of the NHS would be in doubt. The clause is amended – but to what real effect no one can say. Mike Dixon, Chairman of the College of Medicine, concluded rather forlornly that the whole argument seemed "more abstract than real".

Or take the debate about the role of the market and the private sector. In March 2011, at the Save Our NHS rally in Westminster Hall, Andy Burnham, the opposition health spokesperson said: "We are facing a bill that breaks 63 years of NHS history. It legislates for a free market; no longer 'One NHS' but hospital pitted against hospital, doctor against doctor."

Listening to him, you might have got the impression that he would never countenance competition and private sector involvement in the NHS. Yet the Labour manifesto that he had campaigned for not long before promised that patients would "have the right, in law, to choose from any provider who meets NHS standards of quality" – in other words, that there would be a free market and competition from the private.

This is not to say the main parties are identical. There are some important differences between the approach of the last Labour government and the approach of the current Coalition: different views about the speed of change and the mechanisms used to bring it about. Also, there are some serious disagreements about the way in which the current reforms have been enacted and the degree to which they have imposed unnecessary costs and disruption on the NHS. But the direction of travel in both cases is the same.

The real disagreement is not between right and left, but between the political elite and the rest of the population. The politicians and their advisers believe that the system is broken and needs fixing. They largely agree about the way in which it is broken and they agree that we are failing to address the problem fast enough. There are some differences about the merits of different proposed solutions. But on the big questions, they are agreed. The people who do not agree with this view are a large proportion of those who work in the NHS and most of the rest of the country.

It is an astonishing divide. For the past twenty years, the corridors of the Department of Health have thronged with people who believe that greater private provision is what the NHS needs, yet step outside and start polling the public and you struggle to find people who express any degree of enthusiasm for the idea.

Many of the politically driven changes to the NHS have been brought about through government diktat rather than legislation, so opportunities for wider discussion have at times been limited. By introducing such a wide range of reforms in one law, the Health and Social Care Act 2012 created a debate which revealed the full extent of public anxiety about the direction in which the NHS is being taken.

The divide between Conservatives and Labour is as nothing compared to the divide between Westminster on one side and the hospital wards and GP waiting rooms on the other. The medical professionals regard political inter-ference as one more thing that gets in the way of them doing their job. The public have the choice of siding with the doctors who care for them or the politicians who do not. It is hardly surprising they choose the former.

It almost makes you feel sorry for the politicians. They believe there is a major problem with our health service. They work very hard to come up with clever solutions. And when they put forward their brilliant schemes, the doctor looks up from her operating table, the nurse turns from his duties and the patient lifts himself painfully from his sick bed to say with one voice: "What an earth are you talking about. We're fine. Leave us alone." The politician furiously blusters that something must be done. But the public are left unimpressed.

At the Euston Road rally, a young man is sitting next to me who has come into the meeting late. He tells me he is a psychiatrist working in a secure mental health unit in London. I ask him what he thinks of the meeting. He is unsure. He has read Allyson Pollock, one of the most vitriolic opponents of private companies being involved in healthcare. He is troubled by what is happening with the new act. But looking round the room he is worried. "Do you get the impression this is a movement that is growing or ...?" He pauses.

I shrug, but I know exactly what he is thinking. There is a sense that momentum is not on their side. Here is a group of deeply committed people who have the support of the bulk of the medical profession and a majority of the British public. Surely nothing can stop them. But somehow the room is heavy with the feeling that this is a losing team, a sense that this whole debate is a side show and that the real action is happening far from here.

The arguments and theories put forward with such vehemence do not seem to offer an adequate account of why the politicians keep ignoring their demands. The proposals for action to halt the tide of reform sound too puny to constitute any real challenge. There are plenty of strong opinions about what should *not* happen to the NHS but rather less is said about what *should* happen. I am left with a sense that the real forces determining the future of our health service are not to be found in this room or in the fag-end of the political fighting over the Health and Social Care Act but somewhere else entirely.

CHAPTER 2

Going about it like the Greeks

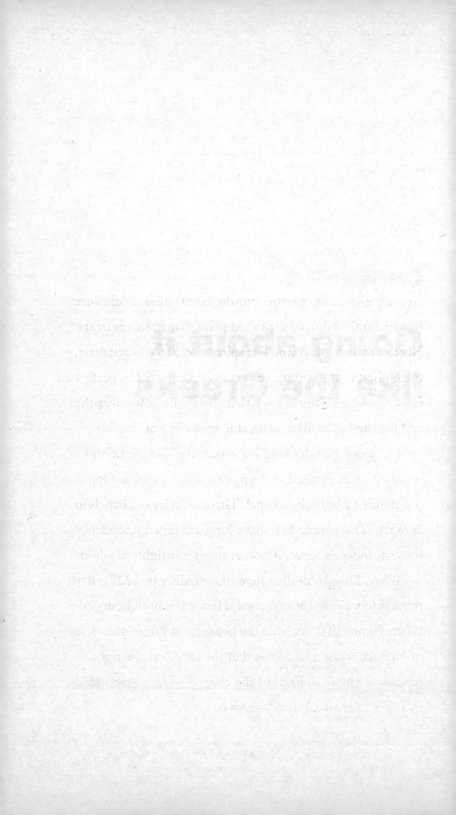

Newark sits close to the Nottinghamshire–Lincolnshire border on the edge of the broad plain that stretches to the North Sea and the Wash. The spire of St Mary Magdalene, the highest in the county, towers over the flat fields, perfect for growing the sugar beet that made the town wealthy and for the US air base that came with the war.

The door I am looking for is near the end of the short street of brick-fronted two-up, two-down houses. Opposite stands a Methodist chapel. There are a lot of chapels in Newark. The people here have long exhibited a tendency towards independence, if not, at times, outright rebellion.

When King John died here of dysentery in 1227, they refused to yield to his successor, Henry III, until besieged. When Henry VIII declared the break from Rome, the vicar of Newark refused to accept that the king had the right to replace the pope as head of the church. Henry responded by having the vicar's head removed.

I knock on the door and a voice from inside asks who is there. I answer and a tall man in dark glasses opens the door, standing well back to let me through his living room and into the kitchen at the back. He tells his guide dog to settle down and follows me through. He sits next to me, turned at an angle to the table, his elbows on his knees, his face towards the floor, listening closely.

Andrew McAneney is a large, physically strong 47-year-old. His hair is cut short – short enough for the scars on the back of his skull to be visible. He worked as a farm labourer until he lost the sight in one eye at the age of 16. He had wanted to join the army, but "that wasn't going to happen with one eye". Instead he worked as a barman in London until he lost the sight in his second eye at the age of 30.

He talks in an even Nottinghamshire voice without unnecessary recourse to emotion. He is level-headed, practical, knows how to take the initiative. When he went blind he got interested in judo. It is one of the few sports that a blind person can play on even terms with the sighted. You just start with your hands gripping your opponent's suit and go from there. He tells me that he has only ever fought sighted opponents.

He was offered an opportunity to train with the British Olympic team. But his partner Donna does not drive and so the travel arrangements proved too complicated and he had to let the opportunity go. He has now had to give up the judo completely after the latest operation on his brain. A blow to the wrong part of his skull could be fatal. He says with a shrug he will have to find something else do now.

Across the table from me sits Marie, the wife of Andrew's best friend. She is petite and well turned out, in a black and white spotted blouse, her dark hair in a neat bob. She has a large file in front of her cataloguing nearly 18 months of correspondence with their local NHS.

"If I didn't have her helping me I'd be lost," says Andrew. "When you complain they are not looking at the complaint properly. They are not understanding it."

"I worry that if you had no one to help you, you wouldn't stand a chance," she says.

Andrew has a rare condition called Von Hippel–Lindau syndrome. This is a genetic condition caused by a fault on the third chromosome that produces tumours along the spine as well as in the kidneys, eyes and brain. The tumours grow at different speeds which vary over time. Because of their location they lead in time to pain, blindness, brain damage and death.

The first Andrew knew about it was when he got spots in front of his right eye as a teenager. He was referred to

Queen's Medical Centre in Nottingham. The condition worsened and he lost the use of his right eye. "Back then it was called something else," he says. "It wasn't so well understood."

It was so little understood that, at the time, Andrew did not make any connection with his dad who was also affected by the condition. His dad had suffered from kidney problems but in the end "it was the brain tumours that got him", says Andrew.

Today, much more is known about the condition and its devastating impact is clear: "My brother died at 32, when I was 30. He had it in his eyes and was blind. But he died of MRSA, in hospital after an operation to remove a brain tumour. That's what took him out."

One of Andrew's sisters also has poor sight and has had a brain op to remove a tumour. She was in Australia when the symptoms first appeared. "The Australian surgeon said let nature take its course. She went straight back to Leeds for treatment," he says.

"My other sister is clear. They can tell from blood tests," he explains. He believes his niece and nephew have also escaped the condition.

Looking back he can see a consistent pattern in his family's history. They were all with the same GP practice – Andrew has now moved – but the GP had little interest in or knowledge of the condition.

"I did say to my GP, should I be screened? You need to be screened regularly but no one was interested. They took blood tests," he says, but this is not enough.

His GP did refer him for an MRI scan – ideally it should happen every six months – but Andrew, who suffers from claustrophobia, could not get into the machine. After he refused the test, the matter was dropped. "No one told me I could have sedation," he says.

With Von Hippel–Lindau, it is impossible to predict when or where tumours will start to grow. That is why it is important to screen for them regularly. If they are spotted in time and are in accessible areas, not too close to vital parts of the brain or spine, surgeons can remove them before too much damage is done. But there are only so many times you can operate.

Twenty years ago that was the best that medicine had to offer. Surgeons would keep operating for as long as they could and then, when it got too difficult, accept that there was no more that could be done. Today amazing things are possible. These possibilities are, in large part, due to the invention of stereotactic radiosurgery.

Stereotactic radiosurgery, like all inventions of genius, is at the same time both astonishingly complex and remarkably simple. Making it work is an intricate feat of engineering; the conception is an idea of pleasing simplicity. If you fire a beam of low-dose radiation through your skull, it will do you little or no harm. A high dose will obliterate the brain cells. Radiosurgery involves sending many low-dose beams of radiation into your head simultaneously from different directions. They are perfectly aligned to cross at one point. Individually they are harmless; where they converge, they deliver a blast of energy powerful enough to destroy human tissue.

Radiosurgery has opened a whole new range of possibilities for people like Andrew. When surgery is no longer possible, radiosurgery can kill the tumours that would otherwise kill him.

In April 2011, Andrew was with some friends in Lincoln. "I got up to get a drink and woke up with blood all over my face". He had lost consciousness and fallen. He went home. "You don't want to go to hospital with a few drinks in you," he explains, and phoned his girlfriend.

Andrew was referred to a doctor at King's Mill Hospital in Nottinghamshire. But, while waiting for his appointment, things began to deteriorate rapidly. Andrew found he could not walk properly.

Andrew was admitted as an emergency to the Queen's Medical Centre again. It took four days to get the MRI done. When it came back, it showed two tumours on the brain and three tumours on his spine, one facing inwards.

The surgeon said he could operate on one of the brain tumours. The other and the growths on the spine needed radiosurgery. He cut out the tumour he could reach and referred Andrew to London to see a radiosurgeon.

This specialist agreed that radiosurgery was the best option. Andrew would need two different operations: gamma knife surgery on his brain and cyberknife treatment on his spine.

Andrew went home and waited. Four months later, when he had heard nothing, he started to worry. The neurosurgeon at Queen's did not know what was going on, so Andrew and Marie contacted their local NHS. NHS Nottinghamshire County said that the request for radiosurgery had been refused six weeks earlier. Andrew and Marie went to see the GP and asked "Where do we go from here?" The GP said he could do nothing and suggested they go back to the consultant at Queen's Medical Centre.

Two weeks later, as Andrew was walking through the park, he started to lose his sense of balance. "It was like I was drunk. I was holding on to the railings and couldn't walk." He was rushed back into hospital and put on steroids. The second tumour had now grown so big that the neurosurgeon decided he had no option but to operate. He was successful but troubled. He said he had been "lucky" going in twice and did not want to do it a third time.

After his second collapse, Andrew was referred again for gamma knife surgery, this time to Sheffield, and finally got the treatment he needed.

Nottinghamshire NHS had refused Andrew's application for gamma knife surgery on the grounds that the medical evidence did not support it. They said his tumours were "asymptomatic" and therefore treatment was not appropriate. The NHS have said they will not pay for the cyberknife treatment for his spine.

Intellectual dishonesty

Andrew still does not understand why his radiosurgery was refused or why, when the doctors had said it was necessary, the local NHS said it was not.

"These people that say no … if it happened to them, would they say no? I know it's not a bottomless pit but it just seems to me that they put money first people second. You think the NHS is there to help you until you are ill – they don't look after any more like they used to."

Andrew is sceptical about the reasons the NHS refused him treatment. Phil Blackburn isn't sceptical – he is certain. And he is spitting tacks about it. Mr Blackburn is Vice-President of the British Radiosurgery Society. He also happens to be the doctor to whom Andrew McAneney was first referred in London.

Mr Blackburn is a stocky, practical man. I have agreed to meet him in a cafe in London but we do not know what the other looks like. His solution is simple. He walks into the middle of the cafe and bellows "Roger Taylor? Roger Taylor?"

Like the stereotype of the hospital doctor, he is public school educated and not one to mince his words. He fights fiercely on behalf of his patients. But there is also a more introverted side to him. He says he was drawn to brain surgery because he found microsurgery was pleasingly "clean and private". Instead of wading around in blood and guts, you are locked in your own world, staring down a microscope into someone's brain and wielding a scalpel with infinite care. Or at least it used to be that way. He points out that today the whole operation is videoed and played back on large screens so that everyone can follow the procedure.

He does less microsurgery now and has special-ised instead in radiosurgery. His days are spent assessing patients and treating them. He deals with a variety of conditions. Most of the work involves benign growths, pituitary tumours, secondary malignant tumours or arte-riovenous malformations (AVMs). AVMs occur when veins and arteries join in the brain. Arteries are strong vessels with thick walls that carry the blood from the heart under high pressure. The pressure forces the blood through tiny capillaries delivering nutrients and oxygen to the brain before it is carried back to the heart under low pressure along the much thinner veins. If the arteries and veins cross, high-pressure blood coming from the heart gets pumped directly into the veins which are not built to stand the pressure. If you are unlucky, the end result is a stroke.

Mr Blackburn's job is to weigh up risks. He says there is an awful lot of information about the risks of treatment. He carefully studies the scans showing where growths or AVMs are sited, judging the chances that treatment might cause damage to other parts of the brain. The "knife" used in radiosurgery is precise but not perfect. There is a distance of 1–2mm from the area of high energy where the radio beams converge to the point where the energy falls to safe levels. When radiosurgery is performed, some of the surrounding brain around the surgical site may be damaged and in this context millimetres can make all the difference, depending on where the growth is located. "If it's in the frontal lobes the risks are lower. If it is by the basal ganglia or brain stem, a tiny spillover and you could have paralysis," he explains.

He also has to weigh up the risk of not treating the patient. This is usually the hardest bit where there is least knowledge. For example, many people have AVMs, and only some go on to get strokes. No one knows exactly what the risk is. To find out for sure, you would have to find a random group of patients, identify which had AVMs and then not treat half of them to see how many of that group then suffered strokes compared to the group that received treatment.

But there is some data on which educated guesses can be made. If you are younger the risk is higher, simply because you have more years ahead of you in which it could occur. And if you have had a stroke in the past you are more likely to have one again.

These situations call for careful judgement and a deep knowledge of the evidence that has built up over the past 25 years. It takes skill to understand that evidence base and apply it to an individual patient. That is what Mr Blackburn does. He uses his years of training and practice, his knowledge of the science and his understanding of the patient in front of him to make very fine judgements that will affect their chances of life or death.

"So I get a bit annoyed when someone writes back to me saying that my decision is not justified by the evidence. I spend my life working on this.... My colleagues and I have had a multi-disciplinary team meeting, we have gone through it carefully, we bring vast expertise – I don't expect some PCT to tell me I've got my decision wrong."

His anger at the system is palpable. He does not believe NHS organisations are being honest when they say they think his treatment is not supported by the evidence. It is a ludicrous claim, he says, as radiosurgery has been a standard treatment for over 20 years. He says it is "intellectual dishonesty". They are pretending to think that because they don't like to tell the simple truth which is that they don't want to spend the money.

"They have created tame committees to claim to withhold funding on medical grounds, when it's financial expediency. They are using the medical skirts of public health doctors to make economic decisions on spurious "medical" grounds. If they wrote back and said we understand your patient needs radiosurgery but we have a limited amount of money and we can't give a kid a renal transplant or a psychiatric patient their day care – well then I'd hold my hand up – I recognise there is unlimited demand chasing limited money – and someone has to make the judgement of Solomon – but they should not be getting their political masters off the hook by pretending they have made a medical judgement."

He says he ends up spending much of his time arguing over who will get treatment with Primary Care Trusts – the local NHS organisations that have had responsibility for deciding how NHS money is spent. In the end it became so frustrating that his assistant, Nichola Button suggested they do a little test. They sent identical details to 16 Primary Care Trusts (PCTs) requesting funding for treatment. Half said yes – the medical evidence supported the treatment. Half said no – there was no justification. The resulting presentation, entitled "The peer-reviewed medical literature varies according to the postcode within which it is being searched", was the first and only academic paper to be presented to the British Radiosurgery Society by a doctor's secretary. Most of the time, he stresses, he wins the argument. But not always.

Mr Blackburn understands why it is happening: "We are in a pretty serious economic situation – expenditure is unsustainable – but we are going about this like the Greeks, we are going to default – all these problems are being built up and nurtured for the future."

Instead of dealing with the problem, PCTs give unjustifiable reasons for withholding treatment. Patients either then shut up and accept this, or try to fight back, like Andrew and Marie. The latter option involves a dispiriting fight with battle-hardened battalions of obfuscators, procrastinators and excuse-peddlers. It is not an even contest.

I ask Phil what he would do to fix the problem. He says he wants more guidelines set nationally on what should be paid for. He and his colleagues are arguing for national standards on availability of radiosurgery. This could help. But he recognises that it doesn't solve the basic problem – that PCTs are finding they do not have the money to pay for the services he provides.

I ask him again what he would do and whether he thinks the idea of getting GPs more involved in managing the way NHS money is spent is a good idea. He is dismissive. He does not believe it will really change anything. I press him again and he answers: "Look, I don't want to get involved in this. I am just a simple doctor. What I want to do is do the best for my patients, not get involved in politics."

It is how many doctors feel. They will go to amazing lengths to sort out the problems of the patient in front of them. But they are wary of trying to solve the political and economic problems that confront the system. Unfortunately, for more and more patients, these are the problems that affect them most.

When I ask Andrew what troubles him most about his experience, it is not that someone took a decision to deny him treatment. It is not that this decision was then reversed after an unnecessary delay. It is not that this delay caused him considerable harm. When he boils it all down, it is the feeling that no one was prepared to take responsibility for his situation.

He is prepared to accept that patients cannot have everything they want; what he cannot accept is that his chances of getting the right treatment are dictated by the arbitrary decisions of bureaucrats and his willingness to fight them.

If he had one wish, it would be that instead of him having to fight the system, the system was fighting for him – that there was someone in the NHS who was on his side, who understood his situation and made sure that he got the best available treatment.

I doubt there is anyone in the country who would disagree with Andrew. It is what we would all like to see. By the end of this book, I hope to have explained why we are very unlikely to see that happen, at least for the foreseeable future.

But before we do that, we should first look at what Mr Blackburn wants.

He, like many doctors, just wants to be left in peace to get on with his work. He wants to be free of box-ticking bureaucracy. He wants to be free of managers second-guessing his judgements. He wants to be free to do the best for his patients.

This too sounds like a very reasonable wish, something that we would all support. But, as we shall find out in the next two chapters, this too is a wish that will never come true.

CHAPTER 3

My kingdom for a cure

In Greek legend, Melampus was an unusually gifted individual with magic healing powers and the ability to converse with animals. He acquired this skill when he saved two baby snakes whose mother had been squashed by a cart wheel. The grateful snake babies licked his ears and enabled him to understand the language of beasts. He is the original Dr Dolittle.

According to the myth, Anaxagoras, king of Argos, decides he needs Melampus' help. His son is desperately ill. Well that's one version. In another, all the women in the town have gone mad. Greek myths generally have more than one version – a tradition that has carried through into the modern era with the Greek government's system of national accounting.

But to get back to the point, Anaxagoras is desperate and wants his son cured. He asks Melampus to name his price and he replies: "One-third of your kingdom."

Anaxagoras is horrified and sends him packing. But, as his child weakens, he realises he has no option. Melampus is recalled and this time he is in no mood for negotiation. "One-third of your kingdom for me, and one-third for my son," he demands. Anexagoras agrees and Melampus becomes king.

The moral of this story is that there is no limit to what people are willing to pay to save themselves or their loved ones from death. This does not just happen in legend. Nicholas II, the last Tsar of Russia, provides a curious modern parallel to Melampus. Desperate to find a cure for his haemophiliac son and heir, he turned to the mystic healer Rasputin. Rasputin's behaviour so scandalised the Russians that confidence in the royal family was undermined. Nicholas, under pressure from his court, sent him away. But when his son weakened, he broke and called Rasputin back again. This story also ends with the loss of a kingdom.

While, individually, we would be prepared to sacrifice an entire kingdom to save our child's life, no healthcare system is going to be able to provide everybody with everything they want. One way or another, there will be a limit to what we can get.

In a market system, the limit is set by how much money you have. That means the healthcare received by the rich is rather different to the healthcare received by the poorest. This is, roughly speaking, how it works in the US. Americans spend a lot on healthcare. As with Anaxagoras and Tsar Nicholas, much of it is spent in desperate circumstances, with the bulk of the additional money coming from high-spending citizens, for expensive cancer treatments and physician consultations in the last months of life.

In a universal healthcare system like the NHS, the amount of care you receive is determined by the system, regardless of your ability to pay. We all accept that this cannot be limitless. No one has ever suggested that a universal healthcare system will provide patients with whatever they want in the way of treatment. That is obviously not going to be possible. However, there has always been an unspoken understanding that the level of care provided is what most individuals with sufficient resources would choose to purchase for themselves. To paraphrase the Rolling Stones: you can't always get what you want, but you can certainly expect to get what you need.

This level of care is rarely explicitly defined, but in the past it has not really needed to be. Medical treatment, after all, is rarely pleasant and most people would choose to receive the minimum amount necessary. In most cases, even if you had a magic bank account that never emptied, you would only undergo those treatments where the benefit outweighed the costs in terms of discomfort and risk. This is what we might term the "money-no-object" level of care.

In most areas of medicine, for most of the time the NHS has met this obligation. If you have heart disease or suffer a stroke, if you have prostate cancer or diabetes, the standard of treatment promised by the NHS is no different from that received by the typical patient paying for his or her own care. Private healthcare in the UK may help you to jump the queue; it may buy you a private room and better food; but the one thing it does not buy you is better quality care. That, at least, is the theory – the understanding – which underpins the NHS.

There have always been areas where reality has fallen short of the theory – mental health, for example. The amount of time you can spend talking to a psychotherapist if you are a wealthy drug addict at the Priory in London is not, in general, something available to NHS patients. Also, private patients are more likely to be able to choose the surgeon who actually holds the knife in an operation. But for most serious physical illness, the care you receive as an NHS patient will be as good or better than that you would receive as a private patient.

This is the unspoken promise of the NHS and for the most part it has been kept. But over the last decade it has begun to fray at the edges. For a small but growing number of patients it has officially stopped being true.

The reason is very simple – the price. The cost of healthcare is rising rapidly and there is no prospect of it slowing. This is a problem that affects relatively few people right now, but that number is growing. The most basic foundations of the NHS are being undermined.

One of the curious aspects of the public debate about the rising cost of healthcare is that the most commonly cited reasons for the problem are not the real reasons. Blame has been put on many things, including increased medical negligence claims and spiralling administration costs. But these have contributed insignificant amounts to the overall growth of costs.

Bad lifestyles – rising rates of obesity and alcohol consumption – certainly add to the problem. But they are not the fundamental issue. Nor is the "ageing population" – the fact that we are living longer and that a bigger and bigger proportion of the population is elderly. It looks as if ageing is the cause of runaway costs because the elderly suffer most illness and consequently receive most medical attention. But ageing on its own would be perfectly manageable were it not for one other ingredient.

The problem is one of success. The problem is not that there are too many old people or too many obese people.

The problem is that there are too many things we can now do to treat their afflictions. If we still only had at our disposal the treatments available 30 years ago, the NHS would not be facing the current level of financial difficulty. The real problem is that these damned doctors and scientists are simply too good at what they do and keep coming up with better ways to heal us.

The speed with which modern medicine is developing is dizzying. Take the gamma knife machines that removed the tumours from Andrew McAneney's brain. They are remarkable objects; operating one is a joy. The patient is laid on a trolley that allows the head to be slid inside a machine the size of a pizza oven. Once the surgeon has decided which areas to operate on, how much power to deliver and for how long, he or she simply presses the button and the machine goes to work. As Phil Blackburn puts it, he can just click the mouse on each tumour and the machine blasts them.

The basic technology for this was invented early in the last century and was used primarily on animals. It was not until 1951 that Lars Leksell, a Swedish surgeon at the Karolinska Institute, began experimenting to see how it might be applied to humans. It took him until 1968 to create the world's first gamma knife machine. When the second gamma knife surgery centre opened in 1985, it was in the NHS, thanks to the persistence of a Sheffield surgeon, David Foster. It was here that Andrew McAneney was treated. The first machine did not arrive in the US until 1987, in Pittsburgh.

Since then, gamma knife treatment has really taken off. Today there are three gamma knife machines in the UK, three in Canada, and 24 in the US. Their use has become standard treatment for many conditions in developed health systems.

Gamma knives cost about £5m each. That is pretty cheap for medical technology. In Pittsburgh, they are already moving on to what they believe will be the next wave of radiotherapy – proton beam accelerators. These monsters cost $150m to build. A 200-ton cyclotron is used to smash atoms and create a beam of protons travelling at a little over half the speed of light. The patient lies on a bed inside a 30-foot high gantry that rotates around them to angle the beam most effectively. A 60-second blast can, it is believed, destroy tumours with much greater accuracy and fewer side effects than current radiotherapy. It is being promoted as a way to control prostate cancer, where damage to surrounding tissue during treatment can cause incontinence and impotence.

In April 2012, Andrew Lansley announced that the NHS would spend £250m to build two proton therapy centres in the UK. A number of objectors have argued that there is not sufficient evidence yet to know whether this is a wise investment.

New medical technologies are both wonderful and terrible. Wonderful because they make it possible for us to cure ever more illnesses and save ever more people from death. Terrible, because every time they arrive, the cost of healthcare rises, making it harder to ensure that the opportunity to escape death is available to all, not just some

The range of things we can do for people has exploded since the 1980s. In the last 12 years alone, the number of adult intensive care beds in England (each of which costs £1m–£2m a year to operate) has risen by more than 25 per cent, from 1,500 to over 2,000. Neonatal intensive care has also grown, as we have learned how to keep ever younger and frailer infants alive.

We have seen revolutionary changes in infertility treatment, laparascopic surgery, robotic surgery, chemotherapy, better pharmaceuticals for mental health ... the list is very long.

Take heart disease, the single biggest killer in the UK. Go back to the 1980s and, in many cases, the best that could be done for the patient was to put them in a hospital bed, monitor their progress and provide them with a limited range of medicines.*

If you have a heart attack today you may be given clot-busting drugs (first brought in in the 1980s). Quite likely you will have an angiogram – a procedure in which a thin tube called a catheter is inserted into an artery, normally in your arm or your groin, then pushed along the blood vessel until it reaches your heart. When dyes are injected into the heart chamber, X-rays can reveal where there are blockages. These can then be removed by expanding a balloon on the end of the catheter – a technique known as angioplasty (first performed in 1977 and developed through the 1980s). This has now been improved upon with the development of stents (introduced in the 1990s). Stents are small metal latticework tubes that can be pushed along the catheter and inserted into arteries, where they expand and hold the walls of the blood vessel open. More recently, these stents have been made with a coating of expensive drugs that prevent new clots occurring. All this can be done while the patient is awake and under local anaesthetic.

---

* This example is taken from T Bodenheimer, High and rising health-care costs: part 2: technologic innovation. Annals of Internal Medicine, vol. 142, no. 11, 2005.

In addition, there is a host of new medicines that will ensure you remain much healthier after your treatment, such as statins, ACE inhibitors and blood-thinning agents.

If you have irregular heart rhythms and are at risk of sudden cardiac arrest, you can now have an implantable cardioverter-defibrillator (introduced in the 1990s), which will give your heart a small shock if it starts beating incorrectly. In other cases, irregular heart rhythms can be treated with a catheter ablation, in which electrical currents are used to burn away those parts of the muscles and nerves on the heart that are misfiring. This is the procedure that Tony Blair had in 2004. It was developed in the 1980s and first used widely in the 1990s.

This array of new possibilities has kept many people alive who would have died 30 years ago. But every time a new technique is developed the cost of healthcare rises. Even if a new treatment proves cheaper than an old treatment, overall costs still rise as patients who were previously untreatable become eligible for care. Every time our ability to treat illness improves, the number of people for whom treatment is a possibility grows.

Heart disease is a good example. Angioplasty is a much cheaper way to repair blocked heart vessels than the previous best available treatment – heart bypass surgery. Heart bypass operations are lengthy and expensive. The patient is put under general anaesthetic, their chest is opened up, their heart stopped or slowed, the blocked arteries are cut out and replaced with bits of artery or vein taken from another part of the body. Recovery takes weeks. Catheterisation is far easier and quicker.

You might reasonably expect that the introduction of angioplasty would lead to fewer heart bypass operations. In fact, the opposite has been the case. The reason is that angioplasty is not appropriate for all patients – there are many whose condition means that a heart bypass operation is the best option. In the past, many of them would have been regarded as too frail or weak to undergo major surgery. But as we have got better at surgery the risks have reduced. The death rate following the operation has dropped steadily as surgeons have improved their techniques and, as a result, people in their 80s and 90s, and those with severe complications who would never previously have been offered an operation are now being treated successfully.[*]

The same has happened with keyhole surgery. It has greatly reduced the cost of operations and made them much less traumatic for patients. But it has also meant that

---

[*] Demonstrating Quality: The sixth national adult cardiac surgical database report, 2008.

there are now far more people who are eligible to receive surgery. So the overall cost has risen.[*]

On top of all this, the increase in the range of treatment options and the sophistication of diagnostic information mean that more and more time needs to be spent making decisions. For cancer patients in the NHS today, multi-disciplinary team meetings are now a required part of every patient's care. The potential combinations of cancer drugs, radiotherapy treatments and surgery mean that for many patients there are literally hundreds of possible treatment combinations available to them. Deciding on the care and making sure everyone involved follows the same plan is a major exercise.

Multi-disciplinary team meetings involve all the key participants in these decisions, who discuss each patient in turn to make sure they are agreed about the planned treatment. They can typically include 15 to 30 different people – surgeons, oncologists, pathologists, radiologists, specialist nurses and physiotherapists – spending hours making decisions and checking they all know what the plan is.

Put these factors together – expensive new technologies, greater complexity of treatment options, a wider range of expertise required and more time needed to manage each

---

[*]   T Bodenheimer, High and rising healthcare costs: part 2: technologic innovation. Annals of Internal Medicine, vol. 142, no. 11, 2005.

patient's treatment – and the number of patients you can treat for each pound spent decreases every year. Then add to this the fact that the number of patients for whom some form of treatment is possible is increasing each year. The result is a much larger bill for doing the work.

The success of modern medicine means that many people are alive today who would have died 30 years ago. This is something to be celebrated. But it is also rather inconvenient. It is rather as if these amazing doctors and scientists have discovered the secret to, if not eternal, at least greatly extended life. Our astonishment and delight at this achievement has been somewhat dampened by then being informed that the price tag is a little outside our budget.

So why don't we just spend more? Surely, it has got to be worth it. We are talking about saving lives here. There are relatively few things that would come above life on most people's list of essential items to purchase. But the problem for the NHS is that what we might be prepared to pay for individually we are not necessarily prepared to pay for collectively.

In the United States, where responsibility for buying healthcare falls more on the individual, people have opted to pay more. Nearly one dollar in every five earned by American citizens is now spent providing healthcare. This presents its own problems for the US economy. Since it is business that picks up the health insurance costs for most employees, business has felt much of the impact. In 2006, higher healthcare costs added about $1,000 to the cost of a Chrysler car compared to a Toyota.[*] In America, healthcare costs are a problem for business as much as for government.[†]

In the UK, where the cost of healthcare falls more on the government, the issue hits the national accounts first and foremost. It puts pressure on the exchequer and on the taxpayer. It creates demands that can either be met by increasing taxation, taking money away from other services or finding cheaper ways to look after people.

The argument to increase taxes and spend more was won by Tony Blair on the grounds that we were putting less into the NHS than other countries. Today the amount we spend is more in line with what is spent on other European nations. But the demand for more spending has not abated and there is no obvious end in sight.

Concerns that the NHS will be unaffordable have been around as long as the NHS has. It was only five years after

---

[*] The North American Automotive Competitiveness Study 2006, published by the Harbour-Felax Group. The figures are quoted in James Surowiecki, Car trouble. 4 June 2007.

[†] See also e.g. Global Manufacturing Competitiveness Index 2010, from Deloitte.

the NHS was founded that the first inquiry was conducted into its long term viability. The report from the Gillebaud Committee in 1956 concluded that spending on health-care was good value and entirely manageable. In 1979, the Royal Commission on the NHS, while raising some concerns, came to similar conclusions.

In 2002, Derek Wanless, a former banker, once again reviewed the financial prospects for the NHS. Like all previous reports he advocating continuing tax-funded services and increasing the money paid into the NHS. But he also identified that rising costs presented the NHS with a real challenge if it was to meet the public's expectation to benefit fully from all that advancing medical technology had to offer. Paying for it would mean changing the way the NHS worked and changing our attitudes to health.

This is the nub of the issue. It is the economics, not the politics, that will shape the future of the NHS. It is the prospect that either we find more cost-effective ways of managing ill-health, or we will find we have to stop doing things for patients.

While the first of these options is preferable, much of what has happened over the last few decades has been the second. The Conservative governments of the 1980s and 1990s abolished free eye tests and dental check-ups for most people. Hospital treatment was rationed by allowing waiting lists to lengthen to the point where some people were waiting years for their appointment or their operation. The rules around long-term care were tightened so that patients who in the past might have been looked after by the NHS now found they would have to pay for care themselves.

This trend has been reversed recently in Scotland and Wales. Scotland has reinstated free dental and optical services and made long-term care free also. However, the cost per head of healthcare in Scotland is higher than in any other part of the UK and waiting lists are longer.*

Cutting free dentistry and eye-care was controversial but it did not undermine the central NHS claim to provide comprehensive medical treatment when you were sick. But in 1999, the National Institute for Clinical Excellence was established to review new treatments and decide whether they were worth the money. Their rule of thumb is that the NHS will pay £20,000–£30,000 to extend someone's life by a year. So if a drug costs £10,000 per patient and clinical studies suggest that it extends life, on average, by six months, the NHS will pay. But if it costs £40,000 and extends life by a year, they may decide not to.

---

* Funding and Performance of Healthcare Systems in the Four Countries of the UK. Nuffield Trust, July 2011. Also, Kim Sutherland, Nick Coyle, Quality in Healthcare in England, Wales, Scotland, Northern Ireland: an intra-UK chartbook. The Health Foundation, 2009.

The calculations are a bit more complicated than this, and involve looking at Quality Adjusted Life Years (QALY). Under the QALY system a year of life spent bed-ridden and in pain gets fewer points than a year of life in full health. But the principle is the same.

The problem with this is the threshold is based not on whether it makes sense clinically to undergo treatment, but on whether it makes sense for society to pay the price. The NHS ought not to pay £40,000 to extend my life by a year because it knows it can achieve a greater benefit by spending the money on others. But I may well want to spend that much keeping myself or my child alive, even if only for a month.

There are then two options. You can let people use their own money to buy the additional care. Or you can try to stop them. The latter is what the NHS tried first.

In 2007, Colette Mills, a 58-year-old former NHS nurse from Hutton Rudby in North Yorkshire, asked that her terminal breast cancer be treated with Avastin, a new drug being used throughout Europe and the US. She was told the NHS would not fund it. She replied that she was willing to pay for it with her own money. The hospital looking after her, South Teesside NHS Trust, said if she did this all her NHS treatment would be withdrawn.

Despite the apparent cruelty of this decision, it is easy to understand the desire of the NHS to prevent the emergence of a two-tier system in which those who can afford it can buy themselves the chance of a few more months of life and those who cannot, go without. It undermines one of the founding principles of the NHS – that we are all in it together.

This may be noble in theory but appears crass when it results in a mother of two with a few months to live being told she will be prevented from using her own money to give herself a treatment she believes will buy her a bit more time on earth.

Collette Mills went to court, as did many others, to contest the rules and the government backed down. Alan Johnson, the then Labour secretary of state for health, announced a change in the rules to allow so-called "top-up" payments for cancer drugs.

This caused a huge degree of anguish in the NHS. When the British Medical Association voted on the issue doctors were split almost exactly 50:50. Many of those in favour of allowing top-up payments would have far preferred to have put more money into the NHS to ensure the "money-no-object" level of care would be available to all, regardless of their resources.

This is why the politicians keep shouting that there is a problem with the NHS. There really is a problem. There is a real risk that we are going to start finding we can no longer afford to be looked after the way we would want to. Or, rather, some of us will and some of us will not.

It is a serious issue, but politicians have been struggled to convey the message. It often sounds as though politicians are saying no more than that it would be nice if the NHS were a bit more efficient. The answer to that is, quite rightly, that the NHS is already pretty efficient and certainly not noticeably more inefficient than other health-care systems.

The problem is not whether we are better or worse than the French. The problem is the same one faced by healthcare systems around the world. Regardless of how efficient they are, the cost of healthcare is rising inexorably and no one is too sure how they are going to find the money to keep paying for it. You can only raise taxes so far. And, much as we want good healthcare, we do have to keep paying for schools and roads and all the other things that government does.

If all we had to do was make the NHS as efficient as the healthcare system in some other country, at least we would know that what we were attempting was possible. The real problem – the problem facing almost every developed economy – is that nobody has yet found the answer. Everyone is looking for a way to ensure that we can all share in the benefits of medical breakthroughs. In the main, that means coming up with proposals to reform the healthcare system.

The French government is equally keen on promoting healthcare reform and is facing equal opposition from the public and professions who remain unconvinced. In 2009, the Sarkozy government's plans to reform healthcare resulted in a far more furious reaction than anything that greeted Lansley's bill. A succession of strikes brought hospitals to a standstill and 20,000 doctors and nurses marched through the streets of Paris.

America has been riven with arguments about Obama's plans to reform US healthcare. What makes his Affordable Healthcare Act contentious is not the idea that every American should have health insurance. It is the consequences of this in terms of the steps the government needs to take to make this affordable by interfering in the way healthcare is delivered – in particular, the creation of an Independent Patient Advisory Board that will decide what government healthcare programmes will pay for.

The determination with which healthcare reform is pursued – and the insistence on the need for it even in the face of public and professional opposition – is fuelled by the belief that if we want to continue to have universal comprehensive healthcare of the highest standard for the next generation and the generation after that, we are going to have to come up with a different way of doing things.

It is a mirror image of what happened in environmental politics. Most people now accept that we will come to a very sticky end if we keep on powering the world by burning up carbon, but politicians were much slower to respond to the evidence than the public. It was only when Green parties started winning elections that the political mood changed.

Healthcare is the other way round. Politicians and economists fear that our current way of caring for the health of the population is unsustainable. But they have failed to convince much of the population that there is a real problem. Most people remain very happy with the way that the health service cares for them.* It is no wonder then if they are mystified by the frenetic activity in government to continually change the way things work.

For those who believe attempts to reform the NHS are part of a conspiracy to destroy it, the arguments about sustainability are either overstated or bogus. Like the debate on global warming, the healthcare debate is affected by the viewpoint of those we might label "sustainability deniers".

---

* See e.g. reports from the NHS National Patient Survey Programme: transparency.dh.gov.uk/category/statistics/patient-experience

The NHS Support Federation is one such voice. It says the claims that technology is making healthcare unaffordable are untrue. In *The NHS@60* it suggests that inflation due to rising drug prices is running at 2–3 per cent a year, a level that is "entirely manageable". While this element on its own might be manageable, the overall impact of rising healthcare costs are proving far from manageable.

Allyson Pollock is another "denier". In her book NHS PLC, she talks of: "scare stories about the 'demographic time bomb' – the idea that as people are living longer, welfare systems are no longer sustainable". In her opinion: "The facts do not support the alarmism spread by policy-makers and government ministers on this score." She suggests that improving medical technology, fewer dependent children, and the fact that older people will be healthier and able to remain in the workforce for longer means that the problem will go away. The attempts by government to use this to argue for reform of healthcare are, she says, "ideological" and "unsupported by sound analysis or evidence".

Again, on the specific point about demographic time bombs, she might be right. Ageing on its own need not result in healthcare becoming unsustainable. But her notion that improving medical technology will make the problem go away seems optimistic. It is certainly not supported by the events of the last fifty years.

These arguments depend on predictions about the future, and all such predictions are uncertain. Governments think it a wise precaution to try to change the way that the NHS operates in order to enable it to cope with rising healthcare costs. But then it might also seem to be a wise precaution to keep increasing the money going into the NHS, at least until we find a solution.

Any real debate on this point went out of the window on 15 September 2008, when Lehman Brothers in New York filed for bankruptcy holding somewhere in the region of $600bn of other people's money. As the world's banking system hit the rocks, taking the world economy down with it, any freedom of manoeuvre with tax funds vanished. Prior to that date, there had been a recognition that something needed to happen at some point in the future. Now disaster was upon us.

In 2009, David Nicholson, the Chief Executive of the NHS, set out the implications of the financial crisis. Health spending would rise marginally above the rate of inflation in order to be able to make the claim that it was increasing in real terms. But it would rise far less than would be needed to meet increasing demand and costs of healthcare.

With costs expected to rise at roughly 4 per cent a year in real terms, this means, in effect, a cut of 4 per cent each year in the money available to the NHS. These numbers do not bring home the full implications. The Department of Health set out the impact of this by setting a target of achieving savings of £20bn on a budget of around £100bn by 2015. That is equivalent to cutting one-sixth of the NHS budget. Imagine closing one in six hospitals and one in six GP practices. That is the scale of the financial challenge facing the NHS. No organisation of the size of the NHS has ever managed to achieve efficiency savings on this scale.

This, more than anything, is shaping the NHS. All of the debate about the Coalition's reforms pale into insignificance beside it. From this point of view, much of the discussion about the NHS bill has felt like squabbling over the beach towels as the tsunami approaches.

Inevitably, the NHS is starting to buckle. When the NHS was last under this level of financial pressure, there was, at least, a very public withdrawal of certain areas of care which gave the public had an opportunity to vote on what was happening. Today, the withdrawal of service is happening in a very different way. A public commitment to maintain the level of universal comprehensive healthcare has been retained but, below the radar, groups of patients are finding that the level of treatment available to them is being reduced.

The people who get hit are those groups of patients who do not have a strong voice and for whom treatment is complex, expensive and relatively new. People like Andrew are first in line to be told they are not going to get what they need. And people like Andrew who do not have a friend like Marie are the ones who end up losing out.

In some areas, the restrictions are more explicit. Infertility treatments are often top of the list of things that are cut back because people feel they can categorise infertility as not a "real" medical condition that should be treated.

Mental health budgets tend to suffer because reducing the level of treatment available to people with mental health issues is far less politically sensitive than withdrawing treatment from people with, say, cancer.

Across the country, local NHS commissioners are limiting access to treatment. In Coventry surgical treatment was refused to elderly patients suffering from aortic aneurysms – a potentially life threatening condition. (The decision was later reversed). In parts of the South East, rules have restricted cataract surgery to only those with the poorest eyesight. In the past, care was rationed by allowing waiting lists to lengthen. Today it is done by commissioners limiting procedures and raising the threshold for treatment.

Faced with a lack of funds, commissioners look to reduce spending. The politicians maintain that, despite the lack of funds, it is unacceptable to refuse to provide treatment on anything other than clinical grounds. And so clinical grounds are found, even if at times they are spurious.

This is the issue driving NHS reform: how do we find a way of using the money more effectively so that all can continue to enjoy the benefits of modern medicine without having to cough up one-third of our kingdom to pay for it? The real challenge is not whether this is a good idea or not. The real challenge is finding something that works.

On my desk, as a constant source of comfort, I have a copy of Random Acts of Management, one of Scott Adams's infallible books of Dilbert cartoons. On the cover, Dilbert's boss (the one with the pointy hair) is holding a spinner that helps him decide what to do when faced with a difficult management problem. The spinner has a little plastic arrow, which, when spun, randomly ends up pointing to one of four instructions: "Yell", "Hide", "Be Unclear" or "Reorganise". Anyone who has been to business school will immediately recognise these as the four primary strategies for dealing with a crisis. Every good manager needs a spinner.

It is something of a tragedy for the NHS that the top-level decision-making spinner kept in the offices of the

Department of Health in Whitehall has for some time now had a glitch, such that the arrow only stops on "reorganise." You can picture the scene. The Secretary of State decides it is time to do something about the rising cost of healthcare. The permanent secretary duly takes out the departmental spinner, developed at considerable expense with advice from many of the world's leading consultancy firms. With a flourish, the ministerial finger flicks the arrow. There is a blur as it spins and everyone holds their breath. Then a terrible groan from all sides as, once again, it stops on "reorganise". They bang the back of it, they fiddle with the mechanism, they inspect it for defects and try again. But to no avail. Every time it comes up with the same answer.

The thing about reorganisations is they give a marvellous appearance of activity. In the face of a public and medical community that are sceptical of politically driven reform, it is easy to understand why ministers might succumb to the temptation to meddle with the one thing that is definitely within their power to change.

But of all the changes that were enacted by the 2012 Health and Social Care Act, the decision to abolish a large proportion of the organisations that comprise the NHS in order to replace them with a whole new set of organisations that only those with the most arcane interest in NHS management structures will ever be able to tell apart is probably the least useful. It has cost the NHS somewhere between £1bn–£2bn in direct costs and countless more in terms of the knock-on consequences.

I do not propose to go into the pros and cons of these different NHS organisational structures as it is tedious beyond belief and, in the end, all such reorganisations have proved remarkably unsuccessful at causing anything to change aside from letterheads and job titles.

Instead, I think it would be more useful to look at what the architects of reform would like to see change about the way services are delivered. Let's take three issues that illustrate the problem. First, there is the role of doctors in the management of health services. The reformers believe that getting doctors to decide how NHS budgets are spent is essential. Much of the public think it makes about as much sense as asking NHS accountants to perform major surgery.

Second, there is the constant drive to close down hospital services and transfer them either into the community or else into more specialised centres of excellence. This is by far the most unpopular thing a government can do and yet there is no prospect of the trend halting.

Finally, there is the desire to get more private sector organisations involved in delivering services. Most of the public oppose it. Most health ministers in recent decades have promoted it.

To those engaged in designing the future of the NHS, these all seem like good ways to improve things. To much of the rest of the population, they appear self-evidently daft ideas that will only make things worse.

CHAPTER 4

Too noble to be measured in money values

In 2011, the National Theatre in London revived George Bernard Shaw's play *The Doctor's Dilemma*. The play is set at the beginning of the 20th century and the curtain rises on the consulting room of an eminent and newly knighted doctor. As the scene unfolds a number of his colleagues call on him to congratulate him and discuss their latest theories.

With collegiate amiability, they dismiss each other's ideas as utterly wrongheaded and insist that they alone have identified how best to treat patients. The joke is that none of them really feels the need to persuade their colleagues of their views because they are all making a very good living peddling their own particular medical miracle. The talk of science is more a parlour game than an issue of professional competence.

At one point, the elderly physician Sir Patrick Cullen complains about the behaviour of surgeons and of one in particular, the fashionable Cutler Walpole. Picture a kindly but cynical old doctor sitting in a wing armchair lamenting how some doctors behave:

"They've found out that a man's body's full of bits and scraps of old organs he has no mortal use for. Thanks to chloroform, you can cut half a dozen of them out without leaving him any the worse, except for the illness and the guineas it costs him. I knew the Walpoles well fifteen years ago. The father used to snip off the ends of people's uvulas for fifty guineas, and paint throats with caustic every day for a year at two guineas a time. His brother-in-law extirpated tonsils for 200 guineas until he took up women's cases at double the fees. Cutler himself worked hard at anatomy to find something fresh to operate on; and at last he got hold of something he calls the nuciform sac, which he's made quite the fashion. People pay him 500 guineas to cut it out. They might as well get their hair cut for all the difference it makes; but I suppose they feel important after it. You can't go out to dinner now without your neighbour bragging to you of some useless operation or other."

The audience enjoy the joke but there is something worryingly smug about the laughter. When the play was first performed, this was edgy stuff – black humour, a strident attack on the medical profession. Today, the laughter is rather more comfortable – a relaxed chortle at how daft things used to be, a joke that can be safely enjoyed in the happy belief that such problems are now in the past.

Shaw himself would like to have agreed that this is now the case. He strongly believed a nationalised health service would end the conflict of interest between doctors and patients in which the doctor's financial interest and the patient's medical interests might not coincide.

He made the point in his preface to the play: "That any sane nation, having observed that you could provide for the supply of bread by giving bakers a pecuniary interest in baking for you, should go on to give a surgeon a pecuniary interest in cutting off your leg, is enough to make one despair of political humanity."

Avoiding that conflict is the oldest question in medical ethics. As Socrates asks in Plato's Republic: "Is the physician – the true physician – a maker or money or a healer of the sick?" The history of medical ethics in the intervening 2,500 years has been, in large part, an attempt to address this problem. Thomas Percival, who is regarded as the father of modern medical ethics in the English-speaking world, recognised that wealth and rank were the objectives of a career in medicine, but he maintained that this must come second to the exercise of "knowledge, benevolence and active virtue".*

Most people who have considered the implications of the influence of money on medicine have come to a similar view. The moral thing to do is put as much distance as possible between financial considerations and clinical considerations. The doctor must rise above any considerations of money.

This viewpoint has, at times, become slightly unhinged. An example of just how far people were prepared to take the point can be found in the writings of the Reverend Charles Coppens, a Catholic theologian from the American mid-west, who lectured on medical ethics at the end of the 19th century. With all the sententiousness of a philosopher priest, he declared: "We find no fault with an artisan, a merchant, or a common laborer if he estimate the value of his toil by the pecuniary advantages attached to it... But in the higher professions we always look for loftier aspirations... [T]he services [doctors] render are too noble to be measured in money values, and therefore the money offered is rather in the form of a tribute to a benefactor than of pecuniary compensation for a definite amount of service rendered" or indeed for an "outcome achieved".

---

* Thomas Percival, Medical Ethics and Precepts, 1803.

To the modern ear, the idea that the money paid to a doctor should be regarded as "tribute" and bear no relation to either the amount of work done or, indeed, whether or not these efforts produced any beneficial effect seems a little naive. But such ideas are deeply embedded in medical culture.

There are many reasons why the combination of money and medicine can be bad for your health. As far back as the Roman Empire laws were passed preventing doctors from taking fees from patients on the grounds that this would mean they only attended to the rich. Money should not be a barrier to getting medical help.

Also, most of us would share the Reverend's distaste for the idea that a price can be put on life – even in a world in which our health system has done exactly this. Even if we accept that a price must be put on life, it is not something you want the doctor thinking about when he has your life in his hands.

Lastly, no one is comfortable with the idea of a doctor weighing up his own financial interests in deciding how to manage a patient. The history of medicine is full of examples of corrupt decisions where the personal interests of doctor overrode the interests of the patient. One of the more spectacular examples was the practice in 18th-century Britain for doctors to declare poorer patients incurable in order to be able to experiment on them. If you were not going to get a fee from them you might as well try to gain a reputation as a scientist by using them as guinea pigs.

This practice so upset John Gregory, professor of medicine at the Edinburgh Royal Infirmary in the 1760s, that he sat down and wrote out, for the first time, a set of principles that could act as a guide to the ethics of the doctors of Britain. Central to his concept was that the doctor must dismiss all thoughts of his own advantage from his mind and consider only the patient's benefit when deciding how to proceed. His other key observation was that doctors should behave like scientists and follow the evidence, not their own personal predispositions.

These ideas formed the basis of today's professional codes of ethics. These codes require doctors to be up to date in their field and to put the patient's interests first when recommending a course of action. These codes have become an important means of protecting patients. For many doctors, the obligation to follow the dictates of their profession take precedence over any other duties that he or she might have.

George Bernard Shaw was not the first person to point out that this form of protection has proved unreliable. Doctors, after all, are as human as anyone else. Conflicts of interest tend to influence behaviour regardless of the good intentions written down in any code of conduct. This has led to the imposition of ever more layers of regulation, from the setting up of the General Medical Council to the introduction this year of a re-licensing system, whereby doctors will have their licence reviewed every five years.

But there is another problem with the traditional approach to medical ethics – one that has only become a problem more recently; one that has been found to actively work against attempts to protect patients.

"Clinical freedom" is the phrase used to describe the idea that nothing must interfere with the doctors' ability to decide what is in the best interests of the patient. There should be no rules governing doctors' clinical practice because they might prevent them from doing what is right for the patient. This would conflict with their highest duty. Professionalism and complete autonomy are the only way to ensure patients are properly looked after – so goes the argument.

This argument has won for doctors a degree of auton-omy almost unheard of in other fields. Even after the NHS took the majority of the medical profession into state employment, it was accepted that to interfere in the way a doctor carried out his job was ethically suspect. In this world of clinical autonomy, junior doctors reported to senior doctors and senior doctors answered to no one but the General Medical Council and God. Once you became a consultant in a hospital you were your own master. The role of the hospital manager was simply to make sure the finances stacked up and the bills got paid. How you practised was a matter for your personal conscience alone.

This culture of autonomy has at its best, enabled doctors to stand up to improper political or financial pressures and get the best for their patients. At its worst, however, it has become self-serving, protecting the doctor from accountability to colleagues or managers.

Just how deeply this idea of clinical freedom took hold can be seen from an extraordinary debate that took place in the 1980s in a series of articles about the rise of evidence-based medicine – that is, the idea that doctors should do what the scientific evidence says works. To most patients, that sounds pretty sensible. But when an article in the British Medical Journal famously hailed this as "the end of clinical freedom"[*] it prompted debate, if not outright hostility from some quarters.

To the lay ear, complaining that your freedom is being impinged by having to do what science says works would seem to display an extravagant degree of self-regard. It sounds like an aircraft designer complaining that his creativity is being blocked by having to respect the laws

---

[*]   JR Hampton, The end of clinical freedom. BMJ, 1983.

of gravity. It stands on its head the very ideas that first underpinned John Gregory's model of what a professional doctor should be – someone who uses science, not their own opinion, to act in the best interest of the patient.

But the medical profession were right to sense that the arrival of evidence-based medicine was the start of the gradual stripping away of their autonomy. At some indefinable date – probably somewhere in the early 1980s – the power and autonomy of the individual doctor reached its apogee. Ever since it has been under assault.

Jim Reinertsen, a US doctor who has thought more about these issues than most people, wrote about this in his essay Zen and the Art of Physician Autonomy Maintenance. He was very clear about why doctors were starting to lose the "unprecedented level of economic, political, and clinical autonomy" they had previously enjoyed.[*] The reason, he said, was that "the public has learned that the basis for it, the full power of our scientific knowledge, is not being consistently applied for their benefit".

It turned out that the rules which protected doctors from undue influence also shielded them from repercussions for getting things wrong. And they were getting things wrong on a pretty monumental scale.

---

*   Jim Reinertsen, Zen and the art of physician autonomy maintenance. Annals of Internal Medicine, vol. 138, no. 1, 2003.

There is nothing new in the medical profession getting things wrong. As Shaw observed, for a profession that prides itself on being scientific, it is at times alarming how firmly doctors can latch on to unproven beliefs if they look plausible.

Tobacco was originally promoted for its health-giving properties. It seemed to make sense. The drying action of the smoke, it was thought, would help fix the spluttering coughs of consumptive or pneumonic patients. For much of the first half of the 20th century, after the discovery of radiation, doctors took the view that it would act as a powerful drug to treat illness. Numerous ways of consuming radioactive substances were devised. The American Medical Association issued guidelines requiring such treatments to meet a minimum threshold of radioactivity to ensure patients were not sold ineffective products. That the products were indeed effective became clear when Eben Byers, a well known sportsman, died from multiple carcinomas induced by his enthusiastic use of such treatments. In 1941, safe levels of radiation were established and were found to be less than one-hundredth of the AMA's minimum threshold.

It is comforting to think that today we live in a more scientific era. However, that cuts both ways. Yes, there is a great deal more scientific knowledge in existence and that has put some useful limits on the territory available for wild speculation. But, at the same time, the vastly expanded body of evidence has increased the potential to act with a cavalier disregard of the facts. It is this latter problem that has come sharply into view in recent years.

Take the example of the use of beta blockers in the treatment of heart attacks. For many years doctors assumed that people with a weak heart should avoid beta blockers. There were good reasons for making that assumption. Beta blockers work by limiting the effect of stress hormones such as adrenaline (epinephrine). They are sometimes used by people who suffer from anxiety as they can stop a racing heart. Adrenaline is used as a medical treatment for people who suffer cardiac arrests. An injection of adrenaline can get the heart beating again. From these two observations, it seems reasonable to conclude that people who have a weak heart should avoid taking beta blockers.

It came as a surprise, then, when studies in the 1970s began to show the opposite. By the 1980s the publication of very large studies revealed just how wrong that assumption had been. Beta blockers were in fact highly beneficial. Patients who have had a heart attack are at serious risk of suffering a second one. But for patients who take beta blockers, the risk is greatly reduced.

Medical opinion had been proved wrong. Fair enough. Nothing new there. The evidence had not been available until that point. What happened next was more troubling. Despite the overwhelming scientific evidence, doctors did not change their ways. Many simply ignored the new information and chose not to prescribe beta blockers to their patients. The result was many heart attacks and deaths that might have been prevented.

Despite repeated exhortation to change practice, by 1998, still less than half of NHS heart attack patients were being prescribed beta-blockers.[*] In 2000 national standards were introduced and heart doctors began a programme to audit practice across the NHS with the result that today, about 95 per cent of eligible heart attack patients are prescribed the medication they need[†]. Ninety-five per cent is pretty good. But it remains the case that some hospitals are still far behind in their practice. For example, in the 2012 audit, the figure was only 78 per cent at Ipswich hospital. In other words, up to 1 in 5 patients had gone home from hospital without the right medication.

It turns out that the consequence of "clinical freedom" is "clinical variation" and clinical variation is not the friend of the patient. Clinical variation is the extent to which doctors

---

[*] JJ Graham et al., Impact of the NHS Framework for coronary heart disease on treatment and outcome of patients with acute coronary syndromes. Heart, vol. 92, no. 3, 2006: 301–306.

[†] MINAP Annual Public Report, March 2011–April 2012.

vary in the way they practise medicine. This can be a good thing if variation reflects a sophisticated understanding of the differing needs of patients. But for the most part this is not what is happening. Instead we find that the result of clinical freedom has been a frighteningly random application of science to medicine.

This is not due to wilfulness on the part of doctors. More than anything it is due to the complexity of modern medicine and the speed with which the science moves. It is extremely difficult for any doctor to remain completely on top of his or her field and to remember to do everything that needs doing for each patient.

But the extent to which current arrangements have failed is alarming. One of the best known studies from the US showed that only half of all the things that would ideally happen to patients, did happen. Only half of the best evidence was put into practice.* That is a pretty low strike rate.

The response to this has been the movement towards evidence-based medicine. This means creating evidenced-based clinical guidelines and telling doctors to follow them. Auditing the record of how each patient is treated to see how doctors are performing has often followed. Publishing

---

* EA McGlynn et al., The quality of health care delivered to adults in the United States. New England Journal of Medicine, vol. 348, 2003: 2635–45.

information about how well different doctors and organisations perform has been a powerful way of incentivising people to follow the guidelines.

These efforts have had some success in improving the reliability of medicine – although achieving nothing like the level of reliability advocates would like to see in large part, because some doctors remain uncomfortable with the implications.

In effect, what is being said is that they are safer if they just stick to following rules. What's more, the only way to make them do it is to record everything they do. To some that seems a little threatening.

The rules and guidelines that are developed range across all aspects of care from something as simple and obvious as requiring surgeons to check they have the right patient in the operating theatre before they start cutting to far more complex criteria for judging whether a particular prescription is appropriate for any given patient. There are now myriad sources of such guidelines and growing evidence of their benefit, but it remains an uphill struggle to implement them consistently.

The idea is disliked by many doctors. Some argue it will stifle innovation. Some find it demeaning to their professional pride to follow what is sometimes dismissively called "cook-book" medicine. Others are troubled by the fact that however subtly the guidelines are written they will never fully capture the complexity of the case in front of them. In some cases the guidelines may simply be wrong – after all, the writers of guidelines are also capable of making mistakes. Being required to follow rules even when they are inappropriate would be professionally irresponsible.

This is a real ethical dilemma. There will without doubt be occasions when a doctor will be able to correctly spot that following a guideline is inappropriate. It seems very wrong to expect them not to act on this judgement. Against this, there is the evidence that allowing doctors the freedom to ignore guidelines when they decide it is appropriate, results in poorer care overall, as they will more often make a wrong judgement to ignore the guidelines than a correct one. That's why the guidelines were needed in the first place.

Despite there being no wholly satisfactory conclusion to this debate, the conclusion of the medical community has, on balance, been to push for standards. It has meant the introduction of more and more rules and guidelines setting out how patients should be managed. As Atul Gawande, the US doctor, puts it in his book The Checklist Manifesto, what the profession needs is discipline, not autonomy.

To the extent that the problem of variation was primarily one of protecting the safety of patients, the medical community has taken the lead. But things have become more contested as attention has moved to the question of money and waste.

Clinical variation and disregard for evidence is no longer simply a question of whether the doctor is doing the right thing for their patient. It has become a question of whether they are doing the right thing for the NHS. Because clinical variation is the biggest cause of waste in the health service.

When we talk about waste in the NHS, most people have in mind the image of a bureaucrat in a suit who has been given the job of filling in forms about compliance with regulations on correct patient procedures or developing an outreach policy for dysfunctional youth. This is not the moment to point out that monitoring of compliance has been one of the most effective ways of improving patient safety in recent years; or that outreach teams have been enormously effective at tackling psychosis in the young. We will come back to the value or otherwise of NHS bureaucracy.

The more important point at this stage is to recognise that, however much waste there may be in the management of the NHS, it is dwarfed by the amount of waste that results from poor clinical practice. This is an issue that separates the public debate about the NHS from the professional debate. When professionals – whether doctors or managers – talk about waste in the NHS, more often than not they are concerned with improving the consistency and effectiveness of clinical practice. When the media and the public talk about inefficiency and waste in the NHS they are talking in the main about sacking bureaucrats.

The problem for managers of the NHS is that to try to influence how a doctor behaves in the interests of balancing the books presents a direct challenge to several centuries of thinking about medical ethics. To intervene in the way a doctor practises medicine for financial reasons would appear to run counter to everything that the medical profession stands for.

The people at the sharp end of this conflict are medical directors. Medical directors are doctors who have taken a role – usually part-time – in the management of the NHS and who are responsible for trying to persuade doctors to change the way they behave.

Umesh Prabhu is one of these. Umesh is from Karnataka in India where he trained as a doctor in the 1970s before coming to the UK. He is a short energetic man who speaks with the clipped and precise accent of his home region in a voice as rapid as machine gun fire. His job is medical director at Wigan General Hospital. He is the one who has to deal with doctors who are not being effective in their jobs.

He has a keen interest in patient safety, medical errors, and why doctors make mistakes – prompted not least by his response to an error he made in his own career in 1992. Since then he has worked on finding ways to help doctors get better at owning up when things go wrong. The inability of the NHS to be straight with patients when difficult things need saying is one of his bug bears. Umesh has lectured around the country on how doctors should approach these difficult situations and is very conscious of the unnecessary additional pain inflicted on patients or their families if doctors or hospitals fail to act in an open and honest fashion at these moments.

He also has a very real understanding of the value of money in medicine. "I came from a very poor area," he explains. "I started working in a government hospital in Davangere – it is very different now – but then it was very poor. I had 2 glass syringes and 22 blunt needles. The only antibiotic we had was penicillin. I was the only doctor. I saw 50 babies a day and 5 of them died."

In 1982 he came to the UK and began to work in Bury Hospital where he encountered a completely different world. "We would use 100 milligrams from a vial of antibiotics and throw the rest away. In Davengere we would have used every drop. At the end of my first day, I got home and added it all up. I realised I had thrown away £200 worth of antibiotics." In Davengere that £200 worth of antibiotics would have been a godsend, not a waste product.

It made an impact on him. He says he took an interest in value for money in healthcare back in the 1980s and would talk about it at a time when fewer people were interested. It prompted him to take an interest in management and led to him becoming a medical director.

Being a medical director can be a very uncomfortable experience. At times it has been regarded by doctors almost as a quisling role – carrying out the orders of the managers who know nothing of medicine and understand only the balance sheet. It is not unusual for hospitals to have to persuade senior consultants to take on the job of medical director because no one is willing to come forward and do it.

Umesh remembers that after he became a medical director in 1998, the attitudes of his colleagues towards him changed overnight. Two weeks before his appointment he had been asked if he would be chair of the staff committee. The day after his appointment things changed. "I remember saying to them, come on guys, it is still the same Umesh, I am still your friend." But there was an immediate fear that he was now working for the other side.

It is easy to see why the job is often unpopular. You have to be prepared to challenge your colleagues in a way that goes quite against normal professional conduct. "Most doctors work hard and provide good quality care" he says, "but a significant number do misuse the NHS".

Not long into the job he was asked to deal with the fact that there were 100 patients waiting for more than a year for a joint injection and nearly 200 patients were waiting to be seen by a specialist for their first appointment. He was surprised as a joint injection takes five minutes. When he spoke to the consultant and asked him if he could get the back log sorted, the consultant replied that he would be happy to do it so long as he was paid £1000. "I was horrified and felt sorry for these patients" says Umesh.

The NHS will sometimes pay doctors overtime or private surgery rates to carry out operations for patients who have been waiting a long time. It is sometimes the only thing to do. But it can create a real financial conflict of interest for the doctor. Treat patients faster, or get paid more if you do not.

The more Umesh looked into it the more problems he uncovered. There were four orthopaedic surgeons, with comparable responsibilities, but vast differences in levels of activity. Two of them were treating less than half the number of patients that the others were treating. He called in external experts to confirm his view of what was going on and found that the operating theatres were only being used for 45 per cent of the time they were booked.

He was particularly troubled when colleagues tried to dissuade him from pursuing the issue, suggesting that it was a waste of everyone's time. With the full support of the

Board behind him, he was able to get his way, but it did not happen without dismissing people, issuing final warnings and fulfilling all the worst fears of those colleagues who shunned him after he took on the job.

In the context of a £100bn health service, rooting out doctors who are performing poorly and wasting a few tens or even thousands of pounds may seem to be missing the big picture. But when you remember that people like Andrew McAneney are being refused treatment that costs £12,000, you quickly realise that this is the big picture.

Doing what Umesh does can be emotionally exhausting – more so even than dealing with patients. Doctors are intelligent, they are on the whole proud of what they do and they do not take being challenged lightly.

The problem is that doctors feel profoundly uncomfortable when someone starts telling them what to do. No one likes being told what to do. But most of us work in an environment where the need for someone to be in charge and direct the work of others is generally recognised and a system for enabling this to happen without personal conflict or animus has been well established over many years. Medicine has done the opposite. Medicine has established a long and venerable tradition based on the idea that no one gets to tell a doctor what to do. Such ideas are the very foundation stones of medical ethics.

When Umesh tries to tell a doctor to change what he is doing, there is a real question about the moral legitimacy of such an action and whether he is preventing a doctor from doing what he or she regards as being in the patient's best interest.

These problems are magnified tenfold when people in the NHS start issuing guidelines to doctors that claim to be based on the scientific evidence and which are designed to stop them offering particular treatments to patients. Now every negative button is being pressed. These are rules based on financial considerations that are being used to influence the doctor. These are guidelines drawn up by committees far from the consulting room, sometimes by people who may have no experience of sitting in front of the patient and trying to assess their best interests. This can appear to be a direct assault on the ethical principles that protect the interests of the patient. This is a very real clash of cultures.

When, in the opening scene of The Doctor's Dilemma, Sir Patrick Cullen bemoans the opportunism of surgeons who perform useless operations, he picks on one example in particular – the removal of tonsils. Shaw would probably not be surprised to know that over a century after his play was written, doctors are still arguing about this.

Back in the 1950s tonsillectomies were all the rage. 200,000 operations were performed each year. The merest hint of an infection and the scalpel would be out. Since then the operation has fallen dramatically out of fashion. This was driven by the fact that it became increasingly apparent that the operation was of almost no benefit to most of the people who were having it. Often, the sore throat that resulted from the operation was equivalent to or greater than the discomfort caused by the infections prevented. This is a disservice to the patient. Equally, it is a poor use of the time of a highly trained surgeon.

The number of tonsillectomies has now dropped to about 50,000 a year. Much of this reduction has been the result of NHS organisations saying they will not pay for the operation. It has prompted a good deal of debate among doctors and that debate illustrates how difficult it is to turn scientific evidence into an irrefutable argument for changing practice.

It has been argued that patients may prefer to have an operation and the certainty of a sore throat afterwards to the unpredictability of suffering from an equivalent sore throat at some indeterminate point in the future. It is a pretty thin argument, but it has been made. For some patients the benefits of the operation may be more than simply avoiding a sore throat – for example, it has been suggested it may help in reducing sleep disruptions caused by breathing difficulties.

These arguments do not directly refute the evidence. They are all reasons why simplistic interpretation of the evidence could have negative consequences for patients. They are all reasons why the clinical freedom of the doctor to decide what is in the patient's best interests cannot simply be over-ridden because an academic study suggests that, on average, patients are not benefiting from a treatment.

The medical profession has not been shy of standing its ground. When, in some parts of the country, rules have been issued stopping the provision of certain treatments the response from the clinical community has been clear, with the Royal College of Surgeons stating that such rules will result in patients being denied vital treatments.

There is a real tension here. On the one hand, doctors have been taught that they should not think about the financial implications when deciding what they do for patients. On the other, if somebody else does this and comes up with the view that a particular treatment is poor value for money, it can be equally problematic.

At the root of the problem is a contradiction in the traditional code of medical ethics – the requirement that the doctor think primarily of the interests of the patient in front of them can be damaging to the interests of the patient not in front of them.

The principle was defensible in an era when the NHS aimed to provide a "money-no-object" level of care for all citizens. But when that promise has been abandoned, it starts to become untenable. Insisting on being free to carry on practices of limited clinical benefit is fine only as long as the resources used to do this do not result in other patients being denied much more effective treatments.

Rules, clinical guidelines and incentive payments are now used both to stop certain practices and to encourage others. In terms of avoiding waste, it is the second of these that may have the biggest impact. There are, in theory, huge benefits from making sure that patients for whom there are effective treatments are getting them, particularly if these treatments have the potential to prevent more serious illness later on.

But making this happen means interfering in the way doctors choose to manage their patients. Doing that without the wholehearted support of doctors is difficult. But equally, recruiting the wholehearted support of doctors for the task has also proved difficult.

The desire to get doctors more involved in deciding how money is spent is, in part, driven by a sense of exasperation among NHS managers at trying to fix this problem. It sometimes feels as though, stung by the limited trust that many clinicians have in the ability of NHS managers to make sensible decisions about how NHS resources and their time should be spent, the managers have thrown their hands in the air and said: "All right then, if you're so smart, you do it."

The original intention behind the Health and Social Care Act was that the bulk of decisions about NHS spending – up to £80bn – would be handed over to GPs. The extent to which this idea will actually be put into practice following the reforms of the Health and Social Care Act is questionable, but the idea still causes consternation in the medical community.

Some are enthusiastic, some loathe it. Many hospital doctors were appalled at the prospect of GPs being given so much power, questioning whether they had the necessary knowledge. Many GPs were equally horrified, quickly confessing to feeling utterly unable to do the job.

The public are equally divided. When doctors like Phil Blackburn say they just want to get on with their job and not have to worry about the money, people sympathise. There is a fear that putting doctors in charge of the money will violate the basic trust that exists between a doctor and a patient.

Clare Gerada, the President of the Royal College of General Practitioners and one of the most fervent opponents of the idea says: "The problem here is not placing GPs at the heart of commissioning, it's allowing commissioning to compromise a GP's responsibility towards their patients."

She believes there should be a clear distinction between decisions about what the NHS will pay for – which should be taken by parliament – and decisions about what treatment should be provided to a particular patient. GPs should not be expected to make decisions about the former as they lack the political authority to do so.

In a speech at the Nuffield Trust* she said: "We mustn't allow ourselves to be compromised. Our first responsibility must be to the patient in front of us. Our next is to the patients in the waiting room. After that comes our responsibility to those on our list. And then to our local community, and finally the wider population. In that order."

In her view: "Being a good GP is not about choosing between the best interests of our patients and those of the nation's purse."

This approach makes sense where it is possible to neatly separate decisions about what the NHS would pay for from decisions about what is right for a particular patient. The difficulty occurs when things do not break down that

---

* The Nuffield Trust and the Royal College of Surgeons of England debate: Could the NHS further restrict the services it provides to offer a core package of services for all patients? 23 February 2012.

simply. For many of the questions that matter, this distinction does not exist.

There will be some decisions about the value of treatments that can be handed to national political decision-makers – about where to set the budget and, consequently, what new treatments or what new drugs are affordable or not.

It is worth pointing out that, wherever this happens, much of the input into deciding the rules comes from doctors. For example, the question as to when patients should get radiosurgery is being addressed by Phil Blackburn and his colleagues have agreed rules for when the treatment is appropriate which they hope to see adopted nationally.

Such guidelines are welcome, but they cannot completely substitute for the judgement of the clinician in the consulting room. Often, the important question will be whether the way a particular patient was managed produced the best outcome for that patient given the resources available – and whether the resources available are being used to the best advantage of patients. If doctors allow these decisions to be completely taken out of their hands, the decisions will be worse and patients will suffer.

In some areas "referral centres" are now used to review decisions by GPs to send patients to a specialist. If the referral centre staff take the view that the referral is unnecessary they can overrule the GPs decision. It is used, for example, to review decisions to refer patients with arthritis to a surgeon for possible joint replacement operations. This approach combines the worst of all possible worlds. The decision about the patient is made twice, which adds to the cost, it interferes in clinical practice and it takes the decision further from the patient. It would be better for the patient if the doctor were able to recommend a course of action that recognised the needs of the patient and identified the most sensible use of resources to address them.

Many of the most contentious decisions are not those taken nationally, or those taken in the consulting room, but the decisions that are taken about how things should be arranged locally. Does Hertfordshire need two neurosurgery services or would one be sufficient? Does London need 20 A&E departments or would 15 be more effective?

These decisions are often even more controversial than national decisions about which drugs the NHS will pay for. But the issue is the same. It is a question of value. Is the money being spent in a way that will bring the greatest health benefit to patients or is it being wasted paying for things that are of little use? As with the other decisions, giving doctors a central role in making them, however uncomfortable that might feel, will on the whole, result in better decisions.

The government has, for some time now, pushed for clinicians to take greater responsibility for using money effectively. This was a policy under New Labour which tried to introduce a system under which GP practices could take control of budgets in 2005. This policy never worked because the PCTs, which had legal control of budgets, had no great inclination to hand over authority to GPs. The Conservative policy was intended to put the legal authority firmly with the GPs. However, in the final version of the Health and Social Care Act this was greatly watered down.

The issue will not go away and it will increasingly affect the lives of all doctors. That is why Phil Blackburn's plea to be left in peace to do the best for his patients and not to get dragged into politics will go unheeded. Medicine now faces a challenge to several centuries of thinking about how doctors should behave. If you go to a medical conference today you will hear many presentations that discuss different approaches to treatment and the evidence that they improve or do not improve the patient's condition. You will hear much less about the cost of these options. This is how it has been at medical conferences for the last hundred years. The doctor's job is to find some way of curing illness. It is then someone else's job to find the money to pay for it.

This was entirely appropriate in an age when most illnesses had no cures. It was appropriate in a time when the NHS did not put an explicit price on life. It is no longer appropriate when most conditions have a great many competing treatment options and some of them are being ruled out as too expensive.

The reticence among doctors to consider the financial implications of different courses of treatment has served us poorly in recent decades. It encouraged the pharmaceutical industry to move their research efforts away from solving big problems towards finding smaller and smaller improvements to existing therapies. After all, if you are just as likely to get paid for making a small difference as a large one, why waste your time trying to find a big improvement?

It has also made it extremely difficult for the NHS managers who are responsible for the finances to find ways of persuading their clinical colleagues to stop doing things that waste money.

Health services are increasingly trying to understand what they do in terms of "value". It is not enough to simply ask whether the patient got better. The question must be: how far did the patient's condition improve and how much did it cost to achieve this? Could a better outcome have been achieved if the money had been used differently? These are the right questions to ask. Are we collectively doing the best we can for patients by getting the most value from the money we spend on healthcare.

If value is to be the measure of good medicine, it must also become the language of good doctors. Today, we have doctors and nurses who were trained in an entirely different mode of thinking and for whom this language is often alien and disturbing. To many it seems downright unethical. But the alternative to coming to grips with it is to continue to behave as if money were no object and to imagine that someone else can be left to deal with the finances; to continue to live in a world in which medicine is "too noble to be measured in monetary value", resources are wasted and patients go without. That is infinitely more unethical.

Doctors are facing increasing challenges to their autonomy. From a world in which "clinical freedom" was the guarantor of patient protection, we are moving into a world in which accountability provides that guarantee. And increasingly that accountability will be couched in terms of value. Doctors will be asked to justify their decision both on the grounds that it was good for the patient and that it was good for the system as a whole. They will be expected to answer to the accountants as well as to the GMC.

CHAPTER 5

Say goodbye to your A&E

Patrice Muamba is a premier league footballer for Bolton Wanderers. In March last year his heart stopped in the middle of a football game at White Hart Lane, the home of north London team Tottenham Hotspur, in front of 30,000 shouting fans, causing a restless and confused hush to fall over the stadium. His heart did not beat again for 78 minutes.

When your heart stops you pass out almost immediately. Within about 2–3 minutes you are suffering serious damage. Shortly after that, if nothing is done, you are dead.

Patrice Muamba needed help fast. He was rushed by the paramedics into an ambulance which then sped away from the stadium as they attempted to resuscitate him. It went straight past the nearest hospital – the Whittington – with Muamba collapsed in the back. The Whittington Hospital is about 4 miles away from the ground. Another hospital, Homerton, is 4.5 miles away. The ambulance drivers instead chose the longer drive to the London Chest Hospital 6 miles away. The distances may not seem large but they can be significant in terms of time when trying to get through London traffic. The ambulance driver's decision added several minutes to a journey at a time when minutes could mean the difference between life and death.

The Whittington Hospital is a big place. Its vast grey concrete bulk looms over the Holloway Road. It has hundreds of beds and doctors and nurses and tons of expensive machinery that bleeps and flashes. It is the main hospital for the people of the area. This was the A&E that Jacky Davis fought so hard to stop from closing.

So why didn't Muamba's ambulance stop?

The reason is, to a large degree, down to one man. If you had to nominate the one individual who has saved most lives in Britain over the past 10 years, who would you pick? Who has done most in that period to prevent avoidable deaths in the UK? One candidate is Professor Sir Roger Boyle, who, between 2000 and 2012 held the post of clinical national director for heart disease and stroke.

When Tony Blair's government decided to spend an additional 1.5 per cent of gross national income on healthcare in 2000, there was much concern about how effectively the NHS would use the money. There is plenty of evidence that much of it went on things that have been of little benefit to patients. But one area where it was used effectively was in the treatment of heart disease.

Back in 2000 your chances of surviving a heart attack in Britain were significantly worse than they were in France. In the decade since, mortality from heart disease has fallen faster in the UK than in any other country for which we have information, but even by 2008 mortality in the UK was still twice that in France. By 2012, for the first time, you were as likely, if not more likely, to survive a heart attack in London as you were in Paris.

This took a lot of investment in new kit, new nurses and new doctors. But the most important thing was not deciding where to invest. It was deciding where not to invest.

When Roger Boyle started work as clinical national director, pretty well every hospital in the country with an A&E department attempted to treat people suffering from heart attacks or cardiac arrest. The result was not just that overall mortality rates were high, but that in some hospitals they were exceptionally high.

Today, in some parts of the country, if you walk into your local hospital suffering from a heart attack, the first thing they will do is take you somewhere else. The reason is that providing people with the best possible treatment takes a lot of skill and a lot of complex technology. Making this available in every hospital is a bad idea. In part this is because it would waste a great deal of money building facilities that would be underused. But, more importantly, it is a bad idea because they would not be as effective at treating people.

The success rates of teams treating heart attacks rises rapidly with the amount of experience they get. Hospitals that treat lots of heart attacks get really good at it. At its best, the whole procedure is executed with slick assurance and military precision. Every individual knows exactly what they should do and when.

If you are lucky enough to have heart attack in Uxbridge, and if you can focus beyond the excruciating pain and the fear that your life may be about to be cut very short, you will have an opportunity to experience some of the finest healthcare the NHS – and indeed the world – has to offer.

The key thing in treating a heart attack is speed. From the moment it starts, your heart muscles, deprived of blood and oxygen start to weaken and die. If you have not been treated within a couple of hours the tissue will be so damaged that you will probably have heart problems for the rest of your life. The target that good heart attack services aim for is to have you into hospital, catheterised and your heart vessel unblocked within 90 minutes of the attack starting.

This is challenging. The first problem is that it can some-times take people a surprisingly long time to realise they are having a heart attack. Once they have called the emergency services, it might take half an hour or more to get you into a hospital. Then a lot of things need to happen. The doctors need to examine the patient and take a history. The paperwork for admission has to be completed. If it looks like a heart attack, an ECG test needs to be performed and blood samples taken. Once the diagnosis is confirmed, it is time to transfer them to the cath lab where the proce-dure to unblock the heart vessels can be performed. The patient is put on a trolley and hooked up to a heart moni-tor. Someone needs to make sure they have a defibrillator and oxygen. Someone needs to get the catheterisation team together and into the lab. Someone needs to get the lab equipment switched on and ready. Once there, the patient needs to be prepped before the procedure can start. There is a lot to do. Everyone knows it is an emergency. People are moving as fast as they can. Everyone is trying their hard-est. But typically it can be an hour or more from the time you arrived in the hospital before you are in the lab and ready to be treated. By that stage, your heart has already very likely suffered pretty severe damage.

That's not what happens in Uxbridge. In Uxbridge, when you call 999, an ambulance will come and find you, put you in the back and then, as they are driving to the hospital with the lights flashing, they will perform an ECG. The ambulance will also have informed nearby Harefield Hospital that they are bringing in a patient having a heart attack. The doctors and the ambulance crews have worked out the routine together, trained together, and they trust each other. The doctors know that if the ambulance crew say it is a heart attack, then they should expect a heart attack. The hospital insists that, at all times, the team of doctors and nurses needed to operate the catherisation lab are either in the hospital or within 15 minutes of it. By the time the ambulance arrives at the front door of the hospital, the team is waiting. They have all the necessary equipment with them. As the ambulance door swings open, the patient is rolled out and the doctor is handed the ECG test results by the ambulance crew. The diagnosis is immediately confirmed and the patient is whisked down the corridor towards the catheterisation lab. The patient history is taken while on the move, and the patient examined as they are being prepared for catheterisation on the table. On average, it takes under 30 minutes from a patient's arrival at Harefield to their heart being cleared and working again. The skill and teamwork required to make that happen is possible because they do a great many cardiac catheterisations. Harefield is a specialist hospital.

But the same results can be achieved in general hospitals as long as they get sufficient numbers of patients.

Peter Glennon is a cardiologist at University Hospital Coventry. The team there have reduced the time from a patient being picked up by an ambulance to being treated by 30 minutes over the past year. He likens it to the way Formula One pit-stop teams work. They have timed every part of the operation to see where it could be refined. When they found that sometimes the cardiologists took longer to reach the ermergency department than the cardiac nurses, they made sure the cardiac nurses were able to immediately begin the assessment. They keep a record of how quickly each patient is treated and share the information with the ambulance crews. When they found that sometimes the ambulance crews were not phoning through to the emergency department until they were on the road, they changed the process to make sure the hospital had the warning at the earliest possible opportunity.

Each of these small changes might seem relatively insignificant. And on their own, they might well be. But together they have dramatically cut the length of time it takes to treat each heart attack and greatly improved the lives of patients.

Glennon points out that an essential part of this service is being able to respond at any time of day or night. If someone has a heart attack at 3am, they need to be treated just as quickly as someone having a heart attack at 4pm. Having experienced staff available 24 hours a day, 7 days a week is simply not possible in every hospital.

That is why, when Roger Boyle began devising a new national service to tackle heart disease he realised he would have to pick some hospitals to be centres for care. Others would have to accept that their role in managing these patients would be scaled back.

He was able to do what he did with heart attack treatment because it involved the creation of new services – rapid-access chest pain clinics and catheterisation labs were set up in hospitals that previously had had nothing of the sort. There was inevitably some debate about where these should be sited. But, since this was a new service, there was little opposition to the fact that some hospitals were getting investment that others were not.

In north-east London, the London Chest Hospital was selected to be the centre for heart disease. The Whittington and the Homerton were not. The ambulance driver with Patrice Muamba in the back knew this and so drove straight there. The benefits of centralising services into fewer hospitals with more expert teams is not just an issue for heart disease. There are relatively few areas of medicine now where the complexity of treatment has not reached the point where centralisation brings benefits. There are now designated centres for major trauma, and if you find yourself mangled after a car accident you will be taken to one of these hospitals, where specialist surgeons, including neurosurgeons expert in head and neck trauma, will know what to do.

Paediatric intensive care units, services for kidney disease and liver disease, HIV services, infertility clinics – all are specialised and centralised. Cancer care is now entirely organised into networks, with hospitals specialising in the types of treatment they can provide.

Care for patients with stroke is being completely reconfigured, with fewer and fewer hospital providing emergency stroke services. In London the number of hospitals set up to handle stroke has fallen from 24 to eight. That might, on the face of it, sound like a bad thing. In fact it is a great success story. The eight hospitals that now treat stroke are exceptionally good at it and stroke mortality rates in London have fallen dramatically as a result. London is now quite probably the best place in Europe in which to have a stroke. It is a poor slogan for the London tourist board but it is a fantastic achievement for the NHS.

This process has, in the main, done a huge amount of good for NHS patients, large numbers of whom would now be dead without these changes. Despite this, there is nothing that causes more outrage and public upset than plans to close local NHS services. This is hardly surprising. The fact that cancer patients today will typically have to visit four or five different places to receive treatment is something that causes resentment and confusion. Most people would prefer to be able to have all the services they need provided at their district general hospital. This would certainly make it easier to get to hospital when you are sick. The only downside would be the rather lower odds of you ever coming back again.

Roger Boyle's particular achievement was to reconfigure services for heart disease and stroke with relatively little public uproar. In other areas, the experience has been less easy. The more common experience is for reconfiguration of services into specialist centres to be met with opposition from clinicians and patients.

For example, take plans to reconfigure vascular surgery services on Merseyside last year. The local NHS came up with a plan to close the vascular surgery department at Arrowe Park and instead send the patients to more centralised services at two other hospitals – the Royal Liverpool and the Countess of Chester. A campaign was launched to prevent this, led by Phil Davies, leader of the local council, and Alex McFadden, head of Merseyside TUC.

Mr McFadden was quoted in the local newspaper as follows:

"The implications of the vascular services transfer are really frightening, not only for the well-being of Wirral people right now, but also for the future. We believe it is the thin end of a wedge which will see many other vital surgical procedures currently available at Arrowe Park Hospital being wound down and sent elsewhere.

"Our fear is an Americanisation of our local health facilities, which ultimately will result in there being one major hospital serving the whole of the region and the rest becoming little more than post-op rest and recovery centres, if they survive at all."

Mr McFadden is quite right to warn that centralisation is likely to continue. Why he regards this as "Americanisation" is a mystery as, on the whole, America's market-driven system tends to suffer from precisely the opposite problem – far too little centralisation and little integration between centres of excellence, local hospitals and ambulance crews. But leaving that to one side, the most worrying part of Mr McFadden's statement is his concern for the "well-being of Wirral people".

There are few things we can say with certainty about this sort of hospital reconfiguration. It is rarely possible to know that one site is without doubt the better candidate on which to centralise service. It is quite impossible to state definitively the extent to which the benefits of centralisation outweigh the risks or inconvenience imposed on individual patients – that will depend on their particular circumstances. About the only thing we can say with some degree of certainty is that, overall, it is likely to improve the health and well-being of the population of the area.

Like heart attacks, vascular surgery is an area of medicine that requires highly skilled teams. If you have a ruptured aortic aneurysm your chances of surviving if you get to a hospital are about 50:50. Around the world, the best hospitals that have specialised in this can get the mortality rate down to 25 per cent. That requires them to operate on sufficient numbers of patients each year. It has been known now for over a decade that smaller units have much worse outcomes. In 2011, smaller vascular surgery centres in England had, on average, mortality rates that were about 50 per cent higher than their larger counterparts. The Vascular Society, which represents vascular surgeons across Britain has accepted for some time that services need to be concentrated in fewer hospitals.

Despite this, the doctors at Arrowe Park fought a long campaign to oppose the changes which culminated in Len Richards, the chief executive of the hospital, resigning after the doctors took a vote of no-confidence in his leadership.

That some doctors often oppose having the services they work in closed is hardly a surprise. However, others have championed the need to change the way hospitals work. The Royal College of Physicians has been running a programme to try to work out what hospital services need to look like in the future. Professor Tim Evans, lead fellow at the RCP for the project has said that about one-third of hospitals should close, services should be centralised and the money saved ploughed back into providing a much higher level of primary care, including access to doctors at weekends and nights.[*] In view of the fact that the membership of the Royal College of Physicians includes most of the doctors working in the hospitals they say need to close down, it is a public-spirited position to adopt.

Sadly, it has had almost no impact on the arguments about hospital closures taking place throughout the country.

Something of a nadir was reached in the Yorkshire town of Pontefract.

---

[*] Shut one in three hospitals says top doc. Guardian, 22 September 2012.

Pontefract is a town of 28,000 people – about the same size as Bicester in Oxfordshire, Trowbridge in Wiltshire or Spalding in Lincolnshire. Unlike all of these other towns, through historical accident, Pontefract has its own hospital. Furthermore, this hospital has its own accident and emergency department.

In September 2011, the NHS announced that the A&E would cease to open overnight as the hospital did not have the necessary medical staff to provide cover. The decision produced uproar. Yvette Cooper, the shadow home secretary and local Labour MP weighed in behind the campaign to keep the A&E open 24 hours a day. There were calls for army medics to be brought in. In January, the chief executive of the trust decided she had had enough and resigned. Two months later the chairman left also. Finally, in October 2012, the trust announced it would keep the A&E open 24 hours a day.

Yvette Cooper called it a "triumph of people power". It would perhaps be more accurate to call it the "defeat of the NHS" – or rather the defeat of any trust in the NHS to act in the interests of the people of Pontefract.

Pontefract is 10 miles – or a 15-minute drive – from Pinderfields General Hospital, a large hospital with a fully staffed A&E open 24 hours a day. Pontefract A&E sees on average between 8–12 patients per night, most of whom are not seriously ill. The cost of keeping the A&E open at night is significant. Pontefract will never be able to provide the level of service that people would get from a larger hospital. If someone in Pontefract thinks they are having a stroke or heart attack at two in the morning and they pitch up at Pontefract A&E they will have made a poor decision that could, conceivably, cost them their life.

Politicians do not say this, because they have great difficulty being believed. Any courage they might have had in this respect was quickly kicked out of them by the events that occurred in Wyre Forest, in 2007, when a similar small A&E department was slated for closure. A local A&E doctor stood for parliament on a manifesto to keep the A&E open and won the seat. MPs were not slow to learn the lesson. Ever since, the one thing you can rely on your local MP to do is to oppose whatever plans the NHS puts forwards that involve a reduction in services at your local hospital, however beneficial that would be for your health.

The Conservatives came to power on the back of a campaign that called for a moratorium on hospital closures and opposed plans to reorganise service in London. In power, their position shifted dramatically when it became clear how untenable this policy was.

The problem is not going away. Plans to reorganise services at St Hellier's Hospital in Surrey were opposed by

Paul Burstow, a junior health minister at the time, because the hospital was in his constituency. In Ealing, 3,000 people have marched against planned changes to services at their local hospital – again, with the wholehearted support of their local MP.

One of the most bitterly fought examples was the opposition to plans to transfer surgery services for upper-gastrointestinal cancers from Treliske Hospital in Truro to Plymouth Hospital. The reason for doing this was that the unit in Cornwall was operating on fewer than 25 patients a year. The NHS produced a number of experts to point out that it was dangerous to run a unit with that volume of activity. Independent experts reviewed the data and concluded that higher numbers of patients were dying than would be expected from a better unit.

Despite this, the campaign against collected over 30,000 signatures on a petition to halt the closure. Eric Parkin, Chair of the local council's Oversight and Scrutiny Committee, complained that the argument for change was based purely on the "clinical case" without considering the impact on the "longer-term strategic direction for specialist services in Cornwall".

I do not think we should be deciding the fate of patients on anything except clinical considerations – that is, the quality of the care in terms of the success of treatment and the experience of receiving that care. The notion that it might be OK to sustain a poor quality service in order to support the "longer-term strategic direction" for health services in Cornwall is troubling.

The problems in Cornwall arose in part because the public were not, at first, consulted about the proposals. But even when consultation does take place, there is often little evidence to show how changes to services will benefit patients. The loss to the local community is very clear. The benefit is not.

Even more concerning is that, after changes have been made, there is often little attempt to find out whether they have resulted in an improvement. There are exceptions. The reconfiguration of stroke services in London was carefully monitored to ensure that it really did improve patient outcomes. All too often, though, an A&E department is closed and nothing further is said. When plans were announced to downgrade the A&E in Newark there was considerable opposition. In Sheffield, Professor John Nicholl, who has questioned the basis on which decisions to close A&Es are made, did some work on the impact of additional travel time on patients. He showed that, for every additional 6 miles travelled, an additional one per cent of patients died.*

---

* J Nicholl et al., The relationship between distance to hospital and patient mortality in emergencies: an observational study. Emergency Medicine Journal, vol. 24, no. 9, 2007: 665–8.

The NHS in the East Midlands has argued that reorganisation of hospital care in the region is needed to ensure patients get better treatment. For example, they have said that there are about 2,000 people a year who would benefit from having their heart attack treated in a specialist centre with a catheterisation lab. Last year only 133 received such treatment. The remainder are given the alternative treatment of thrombolysis and the mortality rate for this second-best treatment is 50 per cent higher.

So the question is, did the closure of Newark A&E improve care for the local population or not? Overall has the change been a success? Without an answer to that question, it is hardly surprising if health service managers find themselves unable to persuade a sceptical public that they are acting in their best interests. They may well be. But if we are asked to take it on trust, most of us will say no. Much as we love the NHS, we do not necessarily trust it to put our interests ahead of its own. There is no confidence that the money taken away by the NHS when a service is closed will be used to provide something else equally good or better.

Across most of the country now, the NHS is planning to reduce the availability of local hospital services. The deal is that the money saved will be used to ensure that specialist centres can deliver the very best care and that local primary care services will be improved to ensure that far fewer patients ever have to go to hospital.

There is a plausible enough theory behind the plan. But the evidence to support the case for specific changes in services is often thin. The supposed benefit for the public in terms of more skilled specialist services and better community care is rarely spelt out in anything but the vaguest terms and rarely backed up with convincing data. It is hard to have much confidence in a system that has such a poor track record of demonstrating that it really does know when changes have benefited patients or explaining how the services it is getting rid of are being replaced by something better.

There is a risk to the NHS management in being more open about the success or failure of reorganisations. We will learn in all likelihood that some decisions were wrong. But the alternative of maintaining that all such changes are for the good is not a position that is either plausible or convincing.

In some cases, the NHS pushes through unpopular changes in the face of vocal opposition. In others – such as the long running attempt to re-organise paediatric heart surgery services – arguments and legal challenges have so far stopped the changes. But one of the fundamental principles of the practice of medicine is consent. Doctors require the consent of the patient before they remove a limb. The NHS needs to do more to win the consent of communities before removing their hospitals.

CHAPTER 6

The private life of the NHS

The NHS is the favourite child of Britain's first success-ful socialist government. It was brought up as a "socialist achievement". It is no surprise if its upbringing has left a deep psychological mark. Created in recognition that the market could never provide for the healthcare needs of all, the NHS remains deeply distrustful that the forces of capi-talism may yet destroy it.

The actions of both Labour and Conservative admin-istrations to invite private organisations to take over the functions carried out by NHS bodies has been the most controversial and anxiety-inducing part of the programme of NHS reform.

The NHS has a fraught and complex relationship with the private sector. On the one hand there is recognition that business provides most of the things the NHS uses. As one NHS manager put it, without business there would be no buildings, no drugs, no machinery, no beds, no scrubs

– just a lot of doctors and nurses in a field in their under-wear. At the same time, there is strong sense that this is peripheral to the heart of what the NHS does.

Some doctors feel so strongly about this that they have created a new political party, National Health Action, which campaigns to limit the involvement of the private sector in healthcare. The NHS, they say, "marked out a space in soci-ety where the dictates of commerce and the market were held in check so as to give expression to socially directed goals". It is fine for the NHS to buy what it needs from the market. But the care of patients should never be handed over to private organisations because they do not, indeed cannot, share the public service ethos of the NHS.

The tone of the debate is at times akin to the Victorian debate about sex and morality. The moral reformers of the 19th century, after careful consideration, concluded that sex was fundamentally impure and ungodly. It might be a necessary part of life, but the best thing to do was to try to keep it to an absolute minimum. Any suggestion that there might be something good about it was the devil talking. William Acton, the leading gynaecologist of the era, declared, in a scientific tract, that to suggest that a woman might enjoy sexual intercourse was a slur on her character. The whole business was fraught with moral traps that could only distract one from a life devoted to God.

In the same way, many in the NHS have a deep suspicion of private enterprise. It is thought to be fundamentally corrupt and something that will inevitably seduce one away from the true path of providing a social benefit.

While Victorian moralists catalogued the many and varied ways in which unconstrained sexuality could undermine civilisation, there was the inevitable response. A range of cranks and theorists from Aleister Crowley to Sigmund Freud began to wonder whether sex might after all hold the answer to all of our problems. In the same way, there are some in the NHS who hold out the hope that private enterprise might solve the NHS's problems. The glint in their eyes when discussing the topic at times suggests an excitement generated by the transgressive nature of such ideas.

The consequence is that the role of private organisations in healthcare has become a subject of fear and fascination. The debate is conducted in terms of pantomime bogeymen. On the anti-privatisation side, the biggest bogeyman is the fear of a "US-style health system". In the main this is rather unhelpful. The primary feature of the US health system is that the private citizen has more of the responsibility for paying the bills. In the UK context, that is not something that is under debate. Privatisation in the UK context means letting companies and charities take control of or provide tax-funded services to the public.

Equally, there are bogeymen held up to argue in favour of privatisation – most notably the caricature of the ineffectual tax-funded bureaucrat squandering public money on politically correct activities of no value to the patients or the public.

People tend to fall into one or other camp. A quick quiz may help to demonstrate the point. Which of the following statements do you think is true or false?

1. The private sector is more efficient than the public sector.
2. The private sector does not have the same caring ethos as the public sector.
3. Private hospitals have more up-to-date facilities than NHS hospitals.
4. Private sector companies that pay dividends will be more expensive.

People tend to favour either the even numbered points or the odd numbered points. Relatively few people will agree with both. In fact, the evidence would suggest they are all, at best, wild assertions which the available evidence would suggest are probably not true.

In the main, these statements are born out of ideological belief. The idea that the private sector is more efficient than the public sector is based on the belief that it ought to be so, because surely the demands of shareholders and the market would make this true. But different pressures in the NHS – a combination of financial constraints, a commitment to deliver a comprehensive universal service, and the absence of the overheads created by operating a market – have resulted in a service which, on most international comparisons, looks highly efficient. The answer to the question as to who is more efficient very much depends on the particular aspect of efficiency you are looking at.

The belief that the public sector embodies a caring ethos that is not found in the private sector is similarly ideologically based. In surveys of patient experience of care – across both health and social care – the evidence does not support the theory. Patients report being just as well cared for by privately employed nurses as by those employed by state-run organisations, if not better. There are certainly many instances of poor standards of care in private sector organisations. But for every one of these there are just as many stories of compassionless and incompetent care by state-owned enterprises.

What evidence exists is usually quoted selectively. Unison, the union that represents many healthcare workers, produced an advert in 2012 showing a picture of an elderly woman in bed with a price sticker on her forehead.

The headline reads: "Shouldn't your health come before profits?" and goes on to say: "Official figures show that profit-making care homes are less likely to meet minimum standards on care quality." They did not mention that, at the same time official figures showed that NHS hospitals were less likely to meet minimum standards on care quality than private hospitals.*

The problem with this argument, however, is not the selective use of data. It is the claim that it is a matter of urgency for those concerned about standards of care and protecting patients. Improving standards of care and protecting patients are important issues. The evidence that healthcare often fails to provide safe care is overwhelming. But to anyone with a genuine interest in trying to understand these problems, the question of ownership – whether you are privately owned or NHS owned – is largely an irrelevance. The difference between the best institutions – whether private or publicly owned – and the worst is far greater than any systematic difference between the two groups.

Opposition to private involvement in NHS services is much more deeply embedded than worries about the quality of care they provide or about the profits they

---

* Care Quality Commission, State of Care Report, 2011–12.

might make. After all, much of the private sector in the UK consists of non-profit-making and charitable organisations. Many UK private hospitals are run by charities. Those opposed to their involvement in the NHS is primarily about the fact that these organisations – whatever their legal standing – are not part of the bigger system.

NHS organisations are linked together through chains of command and accountability, they argue, and are engaged in a common purpose, driven ultimately by the democratically elected ministers in the Department of Health who are accountable to parliament and the electorate. Private sector organisations do not work in the same way. Their primary objective is to pursue their own ambitions, even at the expense of the other parts of the NHS.

In this debate, the important distinction is not between private and publicly owned but between "NHS" and "Non-NHS". This can be seen from the fact GP practices are, in fact, privately-owned partnerships. But their legal structure is not an issue because they are fully integrated into the broader NHS.

The NHS is a siphonophore. Siphonophores are perhaps the strangest class of creature on the planet. The Portuguese man'o'war is one. It looks like a single organism – a large jellyfish that drifts through tropical waters. It is, in fact, comprised of a number of different coexisting organisms that are so thoroughly interlinked, it is impossible to see the join.

In the same way, the many organisations that form the NHS have evolved a way of working together so that they act as one. They have common objective, a common language and a common worldview. The private sector is not part of the organism. It is alien, a foreign body in the system, a potential predator and a threat to the status quo. The private sector does not feel the same responsibility to the wider NHS. Its responsibility is to its own aims and objectives.

This is an accusation that many on both sides of the debate would agree with. One side would see it as a negative. The other would see it as a positive.

To understand how it can be a positive, we need to go to India. India has a publicly funded health system – or at least in theory it does. The level of funding is so low that a very large private healthcare industry has developed to fill the space left empty by the public system.

India has a remarkable medical culture. It trains thousands of doctors who work in the UK and the US while at the same time struggling to find ways to provide healthcare affordably to a population of over one billion. The result has been the appearance of some of the most innovative healthcare organisations in the world.

One of the great heroes of this story is a man called G Venkataswamy. He was 62 years old and retired when he decided he needed a new challenge. He had been an eye surgeon all his life, treating many different conditions, but in particular dealing with the many people who develop cataracts in their eyes. Cataracts are relatively simple to treat, but they still cost money. In the US an operation will cost $2,500. In India, a normal hospital will charge $300. But for millions of Indians earning less than $2 a day, $300 is not a sum that they can afford.

Venkataswamy's answer was to look at other industries – for example at McDonald's – to see how they could make things cheaply by breaking processes down into simple repeatable steps. The very idea that medicine can be compared to hamburger-flipping might seem offensive to doctors. But in this case, it proved to be extremely useful.

Venkataswamy looked at eye surgery as if it was flipping hamburgers. He broke it down into simple tasks and trained lower-paid employees to do as much as possible. He standardised the process, streamlined it and made sure the more expensive surgeons only did the difficult tasks that no one else could do. As a result, surgeons employed in the Aravind Eye Hospitals he founded carry out 2,000 operations a year. In the UK the equivalent figure for some surgeons is one-tenth of that. And they were creative about how they organised services. Rural clinics are positioned close to communities that might not be able to get care otherwise. These clinics are able to remotely consult with the central hospitals where more experienced staff are located.

The result is that an eye operation at Aravind costs $25. Aravind has become the largest provider of cataract surgery in the world. It charges some of its patients between $50 and $300 dollars and as a result can afford to treat more than half its patients for free. Tens of thousands of people have been saved from blindness as a result.

Dr Devi Shetty has achieved the same success with his organisation Narayana Hrudayalaya. Its heart hospital in Bangalore has 1,000 beds and carries out over 10,000 heart operations each year. He has brought the cost per operation down to £500 compared to over £10,000 in the UK, and the outcomes for patients are equivalent to anything achieved in Europe or the US. With additional investment he is now setting up similar centres across India and believes that by using economies of scale he can halve the cost of good healthcare.

The publicly funded health system in India is so poor that people such as Devi Shetty and Venkataswamy have not had to worry about how they integrate with the system around them. Indeed, in the main, the role of government has been to remove restrictions that would otherwise have prevented them setting up their businesses. One organisation is not-for-profit, one is for-profit. But both have been hailed throughout India for revolutionising the way healthcare is provided.

Their particular contribution has been to show how new ways of providing care can produce dramatic improvements in productivity and greatly reduce the cost. It is something private sector organisations do well. In a country like India, where the cost of healthcare is a fundamental barrier to people receiving care, improving productivity is immediately recognised as an enormous social benefit. That is not true of the health system in the UK where "productivity" and "care" are more usually seen as being conflicting objectives. We lag far behind India in understanding that improving productivity is the single most powerful way of increasing access to healthcare for all.

The supporters of private involvement in NHS provision hope that the new organisations will produce similar levels of innovation and improvements in productivity; that they will disregard the way that the NHS normally works and challenge it with new and different ways of working. This in turn will drive the NHS to become more efficient in the way it delivers care.

To date, the programme in the UK could not be said to have been a great driver of innovation. The biggest financial involvement of the private sector has been through the private finance initiative, which was innovative because it enabled the NHS to borrow large sums of money without any of it appearing on the national debt. It has not proved effective at delivering services any more efficiently or cost effectively. Indeed, the reverse has often been the case.*

A more innovative programme has been one largely a copy of the approach worked out in India. In 2000, Labour announced a programme in its NHS plan to start creating "treatment centres" – large centres focused on routine surgery that would be able to streamline the process and bring down the cost radically. We are not doing badly. There are over twenty treatment centres in the country currently performing routine operations such as cataracts and hip replacements.

Some treatment centres were created within NHS organisations. Others were created through contracts with private companies. Businesses such as Care UK, have set up a number of these so-called Independent Sector Treatment Centres. Overall 10 per cent of cataract operations

---

* Allyson Pollock has set out in detail why many such schemes have provided spurious evidence to suggest they are cost-saving. See for example D Gaffney et al., PFI in the NHS: is there an economic case? BMJ, vol. 319, 1999: 116–119.

in the UK paid for by the NHS are now done in privately run centres.

The BMA strongly opposed this development under the slogan: "Look after our NHS: publicly funded, publicly owned". The ISTC programme involved shipping in doctors from abroad to compete directly with NHS services. The BMJ published a number of claims that the cost of the treatment was too high and the quality was poor.* More detailed subsequent research has concluded that they have produced outcomes that are better or equivalent to the NHS and patients report a better experience.†

The government's determination to force private sector provision upon a resistant NHS led to some pretty dirty fighting. In theory, local NHS commissioners could

---

* The BMA record on campaigning on changes to health services has been remarkably consistent throughout the history of the NHS in one regard. Whatever it opposes tends to happen. It fought the taking of hospitals into public ownership in 1948. It fought against the introduction of the internal market in the 1990s. It fought against the introduction of private competition more recently. In general, these disputes are resolved by the politicians pushing through the change they want and the BMA using the negotiations to argue for better terms and conditions for its members. The main outcome of this process is that the UK now has among the highest paid doctors in the world.

† J Chard et al., Outcomes of elective surgery undertaken in independent sector treatment centres and NHS providers in England: audit of patient outcomes in surgery. BMJ, vol. 343, 2011. d6404.

decide whether or not they wanted privately provided services. But when the NHS in Oxfordshire decided they did not want a private treatment centre on their doorstep as proposed by the Department of Health, the board of the PCT was threatened with dismissal unless they revised their view.

The contracts were also controversial. The first ISTCs to set up were offered guaranteed contracts regardless of how many patients they treated. This meant that, in their first years, the cost per treatment of patients at ISTCs was far too high. However, over time, volumes have risen to a level where the costs are in line with NHS levels. Ironically, the high initial cost of these contracts was in part caused by the opposition to them. It is hard to persuade private healthcare organisations to invest in creating new facilities if there are powerful voices saying they strongly oppose these plans and will aim to reverse them at the first opportunity.

Despite the arguments, the ISTC programme has been good for patients. It has increased capacity and helped drive down waiting lists. The service provided has been of a high quality and patients report being very satisfied with the way they have been looked after. Also, the fact that ISTCs compete directly with NHS hospitals has put pressure on NHS organisations to up their game. For a medical direc- tor like Umesh Prabhu trying to persuade his doctors to improve, the possibility that someone else might come and take their patients gives the conversation a bit more bite.

Perhaps most important is the fact that the biggest fears of the NHS – that private competition would undermine the viability of local NHS services – has not come to pass.

But have we really seen any innovation in the way services are delivered? The services themselves do not appear particularly new or ground-breaking. Perhaps one thing it has done is raise awareness that healthcare is a business. Like business, it uses resources to provide a benefit to people and it can often help to think like a business. An example of this has been the arrival of "chains" of services and NHS franchises.

One of the rules of business success is focus. Limit what you do and get good at it. Toyota Motor Corporation has annual revenues of about £150bn. It is focussed, in the main, on one thing. It makes cars. It does not even make that many different types of cars with many of its models derived from a much smaller number of basic templates. Costa Coffee pulls in about £340m a year. It does one thing. It makes coffee. When Costa decides to open a new coffee shop it does not spend much time thinking about the design of the furniture, the type of coffee to buy, the best way to make it, how to check the quality and so on. When Costa opens a new coffee shop it can pretty well take the whole thing out of a box and throw it up in a matter of days.

The contrast with a district general hospital is rather stark. A typical one, like Bradford General Hospital, deals with over 800 different types of diagnosis on a regular basis – that is, 800 different processes.* Because they all take place in a hospital we imagine there is much more in common across them than there really is. Delivering a baby, providing radiotherapy, assessing an older person for Parkinson's disease – if it were not for the fact that all these processes take place inside the same building, conducted by men and women in white coats, it would be apparent how very different they are.

In business terms, a hospital is a souk. It is a large building filled with a hundred or so stallholders offering an impressive array of wares. Each stall holder is an expert in his or her own field and often defensive of their way of doing business. Above all this sits a chief executive who, in theory, is responsible for the quality of the merchandise in every one of these stalls.

Bradford General Hospital has an income of about £300m a year. That makes it similar in size to Costa Coffee. Now imagine that Costa was not just making coffee – it was

---

* As defined with healthcare resource groups. Defined by diagnosis alone the range would be even wider.

marketing several hundred different product lines ranging from underwear to jet engines – and you start to understand the challenge a hospital chief executive faces. That things sometimes do not work as efficiently or as safely as they should is hardly surprising.

Compare that with Care UK. It was paid about £60m over the last year for providing services at eight treatment centres. But these centres focused on a much more specific group of patients. There were no emergencies, no deliveries, no cancer patients. Overall, more than 50 per cent of its activity was accounted for by just a handful of diagnoses.

Critics of private sector involvement in the NHS object that this is unfair – that Care UK are being given too easy a job to do while NHS organisations are left to deal with the hard stuff. But that is exactly the aim. Just as Aravind honed the cataract process until it was many times cheaper than the services offered by others, the aim is that ISTCs can find quicker and cheaper ways to deal with the easier patients. One advantage for Care UK is that if they find a better way of doing something they can implement it across all of their services immediately. In contrast, when an NHS hospital comes up with a good idea, it will often remain a peculiarity of that particular institution.

NHS organisations are now starting to adopt the chain model. Moorfields, the specialist eye hospital in London, manages eye care services for 10 other NHS hospitals. It has now also opened a unit in Dubai. Similarly, the Royal Marsden Hospital runs a specialist cancer unit at Kingston Hospital and plans to expand further.

Since 2000, both Labour and Conservative governments have encouraged greater private participation in the NHS. The Labour ISTC programme was centrally planned, with national contracts being awarded and local areas being persuaded, sometimes with menaces, to allow the new services in.

Andrew Lansley had in mind a more free market approach which was to rely on a regulator, Monitor, who would be expected to enforce fair competition. If there was any attempt to obstruct private companies competing for NHS patients, Monitor would intervene. However the plan never made it off the drawing board. There were fears that uncontrolled private competition would fragment the service to the point where doctors' training would start to suffer or key services would become financially unviable. The extent to which these concerns were a real threat or were exaggerated to protect NHS organisations from outside competition is hotly disputed.

Also, there was a risk that local NHS organisations might have been blocked from integrating services in ways that would benefit patients. If NHS organisations agreed to work together in a way that produced a better, more joined-up service, they might have been judged to be conspiring to prevent competition. Parliament amended the bill so that Monitor was required to give equal regard to both the benefits of competition and the need to integrate services.

We have yet to feel the full impact of these changes but we can expect to see more services taken over by private operators in coming years. In 2012 there were a number of privatisations of community services (as a result of changes brought in by the last Labour administration). For example, in Devon, Richard Branson's Virgin Care is expected to take over the provision of community children's services.

Profit-making organisations taking on the care of sick children raises all the worst fears of the opponents of privatisation. What will stop them simply halving the number of nurses, doubling their profits and ignoring the consequences for patients?

The idea that looking after sick people is a potential business opportunity for profit-making organisations is relatively new. Being a doctor has always been a route to earning a good living. Others, such as pharmacists and midwives, have also earned money for their respective services. But the day-to-day care of the sick has for most of history been a labour of love for family or charity. Since the earliest times, hospitals were set up by governments or religious groups to care for those no one else would care for.

Before the rise of modern medicine, hospitals were not really there to heal people. Their main function was to provide a place where the destitute and desperately ill could be housed – along with the dangerously insane and the infectious. A lucky few might make it back out again. But in the main, your first stay in hospital would be your last.

This tradition carried on through the 18th and 19th centuries, with many of the institutions that are today among the world's leading hospitals established as charitable foundations. Then an odd thing happened. As the skills of hospital doctors and surgeons began to improve, people began to realise that the poor falling on the mercy of charity were getting better quality treatment than the rich. People started wanting to go to hospital. In the 1860s hospitals began to appear that accepted paying patients in the UK. In 1884 Guy's Hospital in London agreed to start taking patients in return for a fee of a guinea a week.

The tradition that hospitals were charitable was so strongly ingrained that the implication of this development – that you could run a hospital for profit – took a century to filter through. Hospitals run for profit did not appear in the US until the 1960s, where they grew out of more traditional doctor partnerships. Profit-making hospitals did not take hold in the UK until the 1980s, when an influx of investment saw the development of a growing number of hospitals built exclusively for private patients. It is only in the past 10 years that it has been possible for a hospital to make a profit from treating NHS patients.

This is an important development and the implications of it have not yet been fully worked out. The risks are obvious and if there is any doubt that they are real one need only look across to the US, where there have been some astonishing tragedies.

Tenet Healthcare is one of the best-known examples.[*] This profit-making healthcare company, set up by three lawyers, first ran into trouble for incarcerating patients in its mental health facilities until their insurance ran out.

Then, in the 1990s, the company set up a hospital in northern California which became one of the most profitable in the country. It was able to achieve this feat by treating very high numbers of heart patients with either coronary stenting or heart bypass surgery. The hospital was doing such high numbers of these more complex cases that it qualified for extra payments from Medicare, the US health insurance system for older people. Investors loved it and the stock price soared.

---

[*] See Stephen Klaidman, Coronary. Scribner, 2007.

It took a very long time before anyone realised that the reason the company could do this was because it was operating on healthy people. That at least is the accusation against the company. It is estimated that heart surgery was carried out unnecessarily on at least 600 people, in some cases leaving them permanently disabled. The company has never admitted wrongdoing although it has paid out hundreds of millions of dollars to settle legal cases. As George Bernard Shaw observed, giving people a financial interest in cutting your leg off can have some pretty obvious drawbacks.

The potential for this sort of malpractice depends on the incentives and controls in the system. Hospitals in England – both private and NHS – are paid according to the number of operations they perform, so they also have an incentive to perform more surgery than necessary. The risks are managed to a large degree by the level of oversight and regulation of hospital services.

In the US, a different and radically new approach to controlling these risks is now being experimented with. It is based on one of the oldest ideas in medicine – a legend from ancient China which became a parable for what is wrong with our health system. The story goes that, long ago, doctors in China were paid a retainer so long as their patients were healthy. The money stopped the moment the patients became sick and only started again once their health was restored.

For a long time this has been regarded as nothing more than a cute observation. Now it is being used as the basis for health policy. President Obama's Affordable Care Act (2010) has opened up an opportunity to try the same trick in modern America. It is trialling a system under which certain hospitals and primary care clinics will be accountable for the long-term health of the patients assigned to them. The payments to these organisations will be calculated on the basis of the degree to which the patients' health improves and the extent to which they do *not* need treatment in hospital.

If it can be made to work it could dramatically change the whole way in which medicine develops. Right now, whether you are a drug company, an NHS hospital or a doctor, your pay-cheque depends on people being sick. Your responsibility is to look after those who are unwell, not to worry about those who might one day get unwell. The idea of a health system geared around keeping people well is truly revolutionary.

The difficulty is one of measurement. It is relatively easy to tell when someone is sick. It is very easy to tell whether or not someone has received treatment. Telling whether or not someone has been prevented from getting ill and checking that people have definitely not needed the treatment they did not receive is much harder. To make a system like this work you have to be very good at measuring the impact that health services have on people's health.

But that is something we need to do anyway if we are going to have private companies offering healthcare. It is something the public understands. Although in surveys the British public repeatedly expressed distrust of NHS services being given to private organisations, their views are a little more nuanced than they might at first appear. A thinktank, Reform, rephrased the question to highlight an important point. Public opposition to private NHS services is not ideological. People are just worried they won't be very good. Asked if they would support private provision if the services were better, unsurprisingly a majority said yes.

We know that ISTCs are producing good outcomes for patients because the outcomes and patient experience have been carefully monitored. But how are we to judge whether Richard Branson's Virgin Care are doing a good job looking after children in Devon? How will we decide whether the decision to let private company Circle take over the management of Hinchingbrooke hospital has been successful?

If we cannot assess this adequately, we should question the wisdom of contracting work to private companies.

Conversely, if we can, we need not be shy of harnessing the investment and innovation of private enterprise to the NHS. You may have picked up something of a theme over the previous three chapters. We have looked at three of the most important aspects of the way the NHS is changing – greater involvement of doctors in deciding how money is spent; the reorganisation of hospital services, with many local facilities closing; and the increasing role that the private sector is playing in the provision of services. In each case, the success of the policy hangs upon one vital ingredi-ent – being able to tell when services are doing a good job.

If we are going to ask doctors to spend more time think-ing about where money is producing healthcare benefits for patients, they are going to have to be able to know which activities are making patients better and which are not. If the public are going to be told that closing their local A&E will result in a better service, someone has to be able to demonstrate they can actually tell whether services have improved or not. If we are going to invite profit-making organisations to deliver healthcare, we have got to have a reliable way of knowing that they have not simply pocketed the cash and fobbed us off with the cheapest substitute for a health service they could lay their hands on.

It is very simple really. If governments are going to push through unpopular reforms on the grounds that they will improve the NHS, they have to be able to credibly demonstrate an ability to tell the difference between good healthcare and bad. That does not sound like too much to ask. So it all hangs on one question. Do we actually know which services are doing a good job and which are not?

CHAPTER 7

In the dark

It is 8.10 on Friday, 27 November 2009 and my breakfast is disturbed by a row on the radio. The Care Quality Commission, which regulates providers of health and social care services in England, has just issued a statement saying it has conducted a spot inspection at Basildon Hospital and found serious failings. The news is a little unwelcome. The CQC is only a few months old. It was established in order to bring about a significant improvement on the old way of regulating hospitals – and to ensure that high standards are met.

Dr Foster, the company I work for, is best known for its annual Hospital Guide, which compares the performance of hospitals across the country. At the heart of the guide is an analysis of hospital outcomes and safety done by a group of doctors at Imperial College led by Professor Sir Brian Jarman and Dr Paul Aylin.

I am feeling rather annoyed with the CQC as I sip my coffee. The 2009 Hospital Guide is due to be published the following Monday and one of its main findings is an analysis that indicates serious safety failings at Basildon Hospital. The results have been known for some time and shared with the Department of Health and the CQC in advance. The CQC has gone and looked at the hospital and decided there are real problems.

I am annoyed because I am worried that the CQC's statement will divert attention from our publication. Maybe that is their intention. It certainly does not pan out that way.

Evan Davis, the BBC reporter, starts the segment by interviewing Brian Jarman, who explains how the data on mortality at the hospital has, for some time, indicated problems.

Davis turns his attention to Baroness Barbara Young, chair of the CQC, and reads out what the CQC website currently says about Basildon Hospital. It describes the hospital as "good" for quality of care and gives it a rating of 5/5 for looking after the health of the population. These ratings, he points out, were published only weeks ago and are still on the website. Now a CQC inspection has discovered filthy matresses, blood-spattered instruments and the regulator says it has lost confidence in the management of the hospital. He adds: "It is hard to know which is more shocking – the care provided by the hospital or the high rating it has received."

Barbara Young was probably expecting to be interviewed about what was going on in Basildon Hospital, not what was going on at the CQC. She seems unprepared for Davis's attack and attempts a series of convoluted manoeuvres to try to duck the incoming fire.

Her first answer is to brush aside the ratings published on their website, saying that they are based on an old system that the CQC is now abandoning.

"So the correct conclusion the public should draw from this is that they should ignore all the information on your website?" asks Davis.

Young reverses sharply. The information on the website, she says, is just a high-level summary. It cannot bring to light all the complexities of judging a hospital. The latest judgement from the CQC is calling into question specific aspects of the care at the hospital.

Davis points out that there are reams of information on all sorts of aspects of care on the website including, for example, a score of 13/14 for "cleanliness and safety". It seems hard to square this with the latest statement from the CQC attacking the hospital for poor standards of cleanliness and safety. How, he asks, are people supposed to know which bits of information are reliable and which not? "A lot of people will be losing confidence in the ratings hospitals are given," he says.

Young tries to shield herself with yet another argument. She suggests that the apparent contradictions are due to differences in time period. The CQC ratings refer to an earlier period than the inspection. Davis is unconvinced. Although it is true that the latest CQC inspection happened after the period for which the ratings were given, it seems implausible that things changed so dramatically so quickly. And besides, the CQC ratings are for exactly the same period as the Dr Foster assessments. These two analyses directly contradict each other. Surely it is a bit more likely that the earlier CQC rating was simply wrong. But who knows? Davis concludes with the observation that "we are completely in the dark".

Just how much in the dark becomes clear over the weekend. The publication of the Dr Foster ratings produces a media storm. The Dr Foster guide contradicts many of the opinions of the CQC. The fact that the CQC now agrees that Basildon Hospital is a problem has thrown its ability to make judgements into doubt.

Civil servants are called in to the Department of Health to work through the weekend. MPs at Question Time angrily demand answers. I am ferried around TV studios to talk to journalists trying to make sense of what is going on. Shortly after this, Baroness Young announces her resignation.

The question I am asked is how many other hospitals rated excellent by the CQC will in fact turn out to be unsafe. It is a fair question. The Dr Foster report suggests problems at a number of other hospitals that are considered fine by the regulator. How is it, I am asked, that a group of three academics in a university working for a small private company can spot a problem at a hospital which a government regulator with a staff of 2,000 and an annual budget of £150m missed?

But the most important question I am asked is "Please tell us definitively which hospitals are safe and which are not?" It is an important question and everyone who asks it assumes that somebody somewhere must actually know. They want reassurance that someone is on top of this and can definitively identify where the problems are. The truth is of course, that nobody can.

Well, that's my opinion. The CQC would say different. The CQC maintains that it is capable of telling the difference between a safe service and an unsafe one. If you go to the CQC website it says: "We check all hospitals in England to ensure they are meeting national standards." These standards include the statement: "You should expect to be safe."

I don't think that is true – or at least not in the sense that most people would understand it. In the opinion of the now abolished National Patient Safety Agency, approximately

1 in 10 patients suffer some form of avoidable harm as a result of NHS treatment. This is in line with the levels of harm found health systems around the world.

So what does the reassurance from the CQC, that it ensures that patients can expect to be safe, mean?

This may seem like pedantry – an overly literal reading of the CQC's statement. Perhaps when it says it checks to ensure compliance it means that it is doing its best to ensure compliance – not guaranteeing it. Or maybe it is saying that people should "expect to be safe" in the same way they might expect the bus to be on time. It will probably happen but there's no guarantee.

I do not think this is pedantry. I think it is an obstacle to safer healthcare. The understandable reluctance to be open about our limited understanding of the problem makes it harder to fix. The fact that, for much of the healthcare we deliver, we really don't know whether it is safe or effective, makes it impossible.

This inability matters. It is the flaw in almost all the schemes that are put forward to reform and improve the NHS. Is it a good idea to let more private organisations deliver healthcare? Yes, if it means we get better services more cheaply. But if we can't tell the difference between a good service and a bad service, all we will get is cheap services. Is it a good idea to make doctors more responsible for how the money is spent? Yes, if it means they can identify better ways to use the money. But if we can't tell where it is being spent effectively, they would be better off spending more time with their patients.

When Dr Foster first started publishing ratings of the outcomes at different hospitals in 2001, a senior figure in the regulator at the time encouraged us on the grounds that it helped to uncover the "big lie". The big lie he referred to was the idea that the NHS provided a uniform service across the country; that whichever door of the NHS you walked through you would be helped to find the services you need and that these services would provide a consistent standard of care.

That "big lie" has been thoroughly examined and exposed over the last decade. There is enough information around today to leave no one in any doubt that there are very large differences in the quality of the care provided between different NHS institutions.

But, as if to make up for the loss of this lie, we have come up with a new "big lie". Today's big lie is the idea that variations in standards occur but the problem is under control. The claim is that the NHS, through effective regulation, is capable of identifying where failings occur and addressing them. The official line is that the normal state of affairs is one in which things work as they should.

Occasionally things go wrong, but if it happens, the regulator will identify the problems and step in to fix it. This is not true. And the reluctance to acknowledge this is directly contributing to the problem.

Every so often an event occurs which shakes public confidence in the NHS. Scandals about poor-quality NHS care are pretty frequent. We have one about once every two years. Most of them flare up in the headlines briefly and then subside. Then, occasionally, a scandal breaks that calls into question the entire system.

In March 2009 the Healthcare Commission, the hospital inspectorate that preceded the CQC, published a scathing report about the standards of care that had been provided at Mid-Staffordshire NHS Hospitals Trust over the preceding four years. In response the Department of Health set up an independent inquiry under Robert Francis QC, which asked for patients and anyone involved to tell them what they knew.

Close to a thousand patients came forward with stories. A minority had nothing but positive things to say. The rest had a wide range of stories covering many different aspects of the care they had received. They are in the main shocking stories detailing errors, omissions and neglect that at times verged on the cruel. About a quarter involve patients being refused assistance to go to the toilet. One in six involve the patient suffering some form of physical injury as a result of falling out of bed or from a chair. In one-quarter of cases patients contracted infections. In many cases these infections ended with the patient's death and the relatives only finding out about the infection afterwards.

The most common themes throughout are of patients being ignored, requests for help refused and questions and complaints rebuffed. The results were that patients were left distraught, were misdiagnosed, were misled and, in many cases, came to harm that was on occasion fatal.

Reading both the independent inquiry's report into the hospital and the report of the regulator, the scale of the failure appears staggering.

Most people who held positions of authority in the trust or in the local NHS have accepted that a major failing occurred. They agree that these events were quite beyond what is acceptable – that this was a catastrophic collapse in standards, that it affected hundreds of patients and that it went on for a number of years.

We are also told it was a one-off event. Ben Bradshaw, then a minister of state at the Department of Health, stated in evidence to the House of Commons Health Committee meeting on patient safety:

"This issue of whether Mid-Staffordshire was an isolated incident was dealt with by the Healthcare Commission itself, by the independent regulator, who made clear both in the report and subsequently to it that they went back and did a very careful check of other trusts that had similar high levels of hospital standardised mortality rates and other indicators that may be a cause for concern and they satisfied themselves (Anna Walker is on the record as having said this; she may well have said it in her evidence to your Committee) that there were not any other trusts that gave rise to similar concerns. The Care Quality Commission subsequently confirmed that."

We are then told one further thing: that this problem was only visible in hindsight. Brian Jarman has kept a tally of the frequency with which the word "hindsight" was used in testimony to the public inquiry. By the end of 139 days of hearings it had been used 456 times. With hindsight, it is possible to see just how wrong things went. But somehow it was not visible at the time.

So to recap: at Stafford Hospital there was a collapse from the normal standards of the NHS, which was quite unlike any other situation, which went on for several years, which has has affected hundreds of patients to the point that protests started. And yet, somehow, it was invisible to those involved in the events at the time.

There is something not quite right here. How can something this bad, on this scale, go on for that long without anyone noticing? Surely just the fact that staff had started to refer to the Emergency Admissions Unit as "Beirut" should have been a clue.

Many commentators on the problems of Mid-Staffordshire have been baffled by this apparent contradiction. Here is a failure that everyone agrees is exceptional and yet it is a failure that is not readily apparent to anyone involved in it. This leads to speculation as to why so few people – in particular the doctors and nurses – objected to what was happening. Reading through some of the stories it seems inconceivable that somebody would not have downed tools in protest.

To understand this apparent mystery, we have to understand how the "big lie" operates and the implications for anyone who does opt to stand up and object to what is happening around them.

The big lie requires that the NHS maintain the line that most of the time, in most placess, things are under control and quality is being ensured. By implication, that also means that failures to implement standards must be defined as exceptional events. If it is generally true that patients can "expect to be safe" it must also be true that Mid-Staffordshire is grotesque exception to the normal state of affairs.

The reality is rather different. The desire to put Mid-Staffordshire into a separate box and label it "bad" while all around is "good" is understandable. But it is very unfair on many of the people involved. One reason why the failures at Mid-Staffordshire did not prompt in staff the horrified reactions of those who read the reports of the inquiry was that, in truth, it was not quite as exceptional as it has since been made out to be.

Paul Woodmansey was a senior doctor at Stafford throughout the period when things went wrong. He is mentioned by a number of patients for whom his department provided a haven of professional high-quality care while standards in other wards collapsed. He wrote to the Royal College of Physicians journal saying that: "many colleagues elsewhere have expressed relief that it was our hospital not theirs which had received such in-depth scrutiny. It is difficult for anyone to maintain objectivity in the face of such a media storm, and I suspect that similar instances of poor patient care could have, and perhaps can still, be found elsewhere. There was also no doubt that many, and I hope the majority, of patients who had been treated in our hospital had received good care. It soon became clear that the real position of the hospital in the national league of awfulness did not matter. What did matter was that many patients had received poor care and, for some, their treatment was appalling."* In other words, Mid-Staffordshire was not a unique case. If anything, it was at the extreme end of a spectrum which shades gradually from excellent, to tolerable, to awful.

Questions of scale are harder to judge than questions of substance. We know that there was often chaos in the A&E and emergency admission unit at the hospital. But then many A&E departments have moments of chaos, many of them have safety issues. How do you know what level of chaos is no longer acceptable?

One piece of jargon from the world of patient safety illustrates the point. "Never event" is a term used to refer to things that should never happen. The term was devised to focus safety efforts on those things that no one would try to defend – things like operating on the wrong part of the patient. NHS hospitals have a duty to record and report how often "never events" take place. As this rather Orwellian instruction implies, it is rather more frequent than "never". In the first year of the scheme 111 such events were reported across the NHS.

---

* In Clinical Medicine, vol. 11, no. 1, 2011, p. 17.

Efforts to focus attention on these events have been very effective at reducing their number. However, the fact remains that they continue to occur, with sufficient regularity that they do not on their own signal that a service has become unacceptably poor. Although everyone agrees that these events are wholly unacceptable, those same people would not agree that the occurrence of a never event implies that a service is unsafe. For that there would have to be too many "never events". But how many is too many? How do you spot when the level of unacceptability has become unacceptable?

You have the same problem with avoidable deaths. The occurrence of an avoidable death might seem like a clear signal that a hospital service that is unsafe. It does not. Or at least not officially. Walsall Hospital currently has a big tick from the CQC for treating patients safely. In 2012, it reported 2,693 safety incidents to the National Reporting and Learning Services over a six month period of which 80 resulted in severe harm and 14 resulted in death. These figures are not unusually high.

Preventing these events from happening is incredibly hard and no hospital has managed to eradicate them. The point is simply that when you realise that 80 cases of severe harm and 14 deaths is "safe", it is easier to understand how it might not be immediately obvious to frontline staff when the line from safe to unsafe has been crossed. Because there is no line.

This is the problem – or rather one of the many problems – that confronts anyone thinking of becoming a whistle-blower in the NHS. If you step forward and say things aren't good enough, what is your evidence? By whose standard of safety are you making that judgement? In the absence of any reliable or agreed upon way to distinguish a good safe service from a poor unsafe one, you are going to have a vicious fight on your hands.

The work of organisations such as the Institute for Healthcare Improvement in the United States and the Health Foundation in the UK has done a lot to spell out what makes a safe service (such as having safety as a board priority) and which clinical areas should be addressed first (such as reducing infections, preventing pneumonia in intensive care and preventing blood clots).

However, the work to start to set out what safe health-care looks like has created a paradox. On the one hand, if you go to a conference on health safety you will hear speaker after speaker bemoan the achingly slow pace with which patient safety is being addressed, and point out without contradiction that the practice of safe healthcare remains elusive. On the other hand, if you say that any particular doctor or health organisation is "unsafe", people start shifting uncomfortably in their chairs.

It is over 10 years since the last public inquiry into standards of hospital care. The earlier inquiry followed the discovery of unacceptably poor standards of heart surgery on children by surgeons in Bristol who were insufficiently skilled at what they were doing. One of the conclusions of that inquiry, under Sir Ian Kennedy, was that clear standards of safety needed to be established.

The trouble with that is that it sets up a dilemma. You can set standards of safety that medical experts – and the rest of the population – would regard as reasonable: a level at which avoidable deaths might be reasonably expected to fall to zero. But then you will have to live with the fact that most of your healthcare organisations, if not all, will fail them and people will expect you to fix the situation, which might prove rather expensive. Or you set much vaguer standards, ensure that most healthcare providers pass them and send out the reassuring message that things are under control. That is the route we have chosen.

So we cannot then be surprised if doctors or nurses are not immediately able to spot when a level of safety counts as "safe" or "unsafe". Or if, when a whistleblower claims a service is "unsafe" they are immediately contradicted.

For many, the most sensible course of action is to do the best with the resources available. Medical staff will be conscious of the fact that there are doctors all around the world working in more difficult circumstances than theirs and that their first responsibility is to do what they can with what is available. They will also be very conscious that any queries regarding the safety of the service or lack of resources would be unlikely to be welcome.

In January 2008, Lord Darzi, a surgeon and a minister at the Department of Health, received reports from three US organisations – the Institute for Healthcare Improvement, Rand and the Joint Commission International, an independent company which accredits the quality of hospitals. Darzi was conducting a review of quality in the NHS and the three organisations had been asked to look into the way the NHS went about ensuring standards of care.

The report from the Joint Commission came up with some fairly forthright observations about the NHS, which they described as having a culture of "blame" and "public humiliation". They suggested that the NHS should try to adopt a more open culture of "engagement" and "involvement". Some NHS managers have argued that this misrepresents the spirit with which the NHS operates. Their argument is not helped by the fact that the Department of Health chose not to publish the report which only came to light after a Freedom of Information requests.

The term "blame culture" is much used throughout the NHS. At times people seem to use it to describe a culture in which people get blamed. Just to avoid any confusion, that is not a blame culture. Blame is a necessary part of life. There is no justice without blame. A blame culture is one in which blame is misused and becomes a baton with which to impose authority rather than an aid to accountability. A blame culture is one in which people are afraid to do what they should or say what they believe because of fear of what others might say about them. It is a culture in which people cannot talk freely.

An example of the impact of blame culture would be Witness D, a nurse in Mid-Staffordshire who testified at the first inquiry into the hospital. Witness D was also a governor of the hospital. Hospital governors are rather like school governors, although there are more of them. They are members of staff and the public who meet to review the decisions of the hospital board and put forward views from the local community.

Witness D testified to the inquiry in two capacities – as a member of the hospital staff but also as someone who was affected by poor care. In her evidence, she describes how her father was admitted to hospital on two occasions, suffering from heart and pancreas problems. She says her father was ignored, tests were delayed and medications missed. It reached a point where she was worried for his life. She describes how she ended up breaking down in tears in front of a surgeon and begging: "You have to help me ... no matter how many times I am shouting, nobody is helping my dad." She believes if she had not intervened her dad he might have died.

Despite this, she chose not to speak up about what was happening in the hospital. She said staff were dissuaded from reporting incidents. After the regulator criticised the trust, they felt threatened and nervous about highlighting any further problems. As a governor of the trust, she did not want to speak out in the public governors' meetings because it would invite criticism from patient groups. "You didn't want to be seen criticising your employers," she said. She said the she was worried about "verbal abuse" from Cure the NHS, the local patient group although later, she clarified that she had never actually been abused by anyone from the group. She dismissed some of the claims being made by Cure-the-NHS as being just their "perception".

Julie Bailey is the woman who founded Cure the NHS. She had an experience at Stafford Hospital similar to that of Witness D. She found herself one night in the hospital desperate for help. Unfortunately for Julie Bailey, she did not know a doctor. As events unfolded, that was to prove crucial.

It was a Tuesday night. Julie's mum, Bella, had just had a blood transfusion but she had responded badly and was starting to pant. A blood transfusion, if it is done too fast, can lead to an imbalance of fluid in the body that causes breathlessness and can be fatal.[*] The doctor had said she would need extra frusemide – a drug that helps the correct this. But after the transfusion the nurse had said she was going on her tea break and the night staff would have to deal with it.

By the time the night nurse arrived, Bella was finding it hard to breath and Julie was frantic. "I asked the nurse: 'Can she have the extra frusemide?'" The nurse looked at Julie and told her that her mother had not been prescribed any extra frusemide.

> "I tried to explain it, I tried to persuade her. I said it must be a mistake. I said 'Do most people have it?' She said 'Yes, but it hasn't been prescribed for your mother'. I said 'Can you call a doctor?' She put her hands on her hips and said 'I am in charge.'
>
> "All I could see was the table in front of me. I can see it now. And her face. I had to leave. I would have hit her… That's the last I saw of mum. She died a few hours later. She never got the extra frusemide."

---

[*] Fluid overload is a rare but well-known adverse reaction to blood transfusion. It can be fatal but is preventable through the monitoring of the speed of transfusion and the use of diuretics.

It would be hard to overstate the impact of this on Julie. That dreadful evening came after weeks of spending nearly every night beside her mother. Earlier during Bella's stay in hospital, after her operation, the doctors had indicated to Julie that they did not think her prospects were good. They had suggested that Julie should go home and get some rest. She refused, and believes her refusal prompted the doctors to give her mum a feeding tube.* It had a dramatic effect and Bella recovered her strength to the point where she was ready to be discharged.

Julie had come to the view that Bella was not safe in the hospital without someone with her. But she reckoned that if she looked after her she could get her out alive. Tragically, the day she was due to be discharged, an administrative delay meant this was postponed to the following Monday. Over the weekend she was badly hurt while being taken off the commode at night.† The injury weakened her and led to the decision to give her a blood transfusion, which in turn led to the events on the Tuesday and the

---

* Only about 30–40 per cent of patients who would benefit from this type of treatment receive it according to the NICE guidelines on supported feeding – while about 20–25 per cent of the patients who do get a tube don't need it or are harmed by it.

† See Julie Bailey's account in From Ward to Whitehall: the disaster at Mid-Staffs, which describes the stand-off between her and a nurse when Julie explains to the nurse that her mother was dropped by the healthcare assistant and the nurse insists that she "slipped".

awful moment when Julie fled the hospital in fury and her mother died.

The sense of loss and regret in Julie is tangible. She had spent much of her childhood with a stepmother, returning to live with her mother when she was 12. Perhaps because of the time apart, they became very close. When Julie moved to Wales to become a social worker her mum went with her. When she returned to Stafford they set up a business together.

After Bella died, Julie shut the business and instead threw herself into a fight with the NHS. Her decision was prompted in part by the letter she received from the hospital shortly after her mother died, asking her to get in touch if she had any concerns. It was clearly a standard letter sent to everyone. The fact that prior to her mother's death she had already written to the ward, to the official complaints service and had taken a letter personally to the office of the chief executive did not seem to have registered.

When she called the hospital and reported what had happened, she came away with the impression that no one believed her. To suffer as a result of care that you regard as substandard is painful. To be ignored when you complain makes it worse. To then be disbelieved when you finally manage to talk to someone is intolerable.

So she went to the press. She wrote to her local paper. She was interviewed by the local BBC and before she knew it she had become the centre of a local uprising by patients who were equally appalled by the way they had been treated.

They began collecting stories of what had happened to patients. They wrote to the media, to MPs and to anyone who would listen. And they began to hold silent vigils in the field outside the hospital – a constant reminder that they would not give up or be moved on.

Julie soon found out that she was taking on more than just her local hospital. She was taking on a sacrosanct institution. It was only a few weeks before the first letters and emails arrived. Julie has had her tyres slashed, things smeared across her windows and bagsful of hate-mail from people who regard her as a menace to the NHS.

The low point came after they closed the local A&E at night because it was regarded as unsafe. The state of the hospital had become a political issue. The Conservatives had promised a public inquiry and Labour had refused so Julie had come out in favour of the Conservatives, despite having previously been a Labour supporter. Labour responded by creating a video in which they interviewed local people to ask them how they felt about the A&E closing overnight. One quote included the sentiment that it would be good if Julie died in an ambulance.

So here we have two women from Stafford – Witness D and Julie Bailey. Both have experienced appallingly bad treatment at the hospital. In one case disaster was averted. In the other it was not. But they both know something is very badly wrong at the hospital.

One, a nurse governor at the hospital, is afraid to say what she thinks in public because she fears it will get her into trouble. The other, a member of the public, has chosen to speak up publicly because when she complained she felt ignored. As a result, she becomes the subject of abuse and threats.

The NHS certainly does have a blame culture, but it extends far beyond the walls of its institutions and has its roots deep in our society. In part it is driven by some who regard attacks on the NHS as sacrilegious. But equally, it is driven by the fact that so much politically is invested in the big lie – the need to reassure the public that they need not worry, it is all under control.

Witness D's belief that her superiors did not want her to say anything is well-founded. As Bill Moyes, former Executive Chairman of Monitor, another healthcare regulator, told the Mid-Staffordshire Inquiry: "The culture of the NHS, particularly the hospital sector, I would say, is not to embarrass the minister.

Aneurin Bevan famously said that if a bedpan was dropped in a hospital corridor the echoes should reverberate around Whitehall. He created a system that successfully achieved this. But the result has not been that bedpans do not get dropped. The result has been that, when this happens, people's first instinct is often to silence the noise and hush the whole thing up.

It is a culture that runs from the top to the bottom of the organisation. Even the people in charge feel they cannot speak freely. Barbara Young is not somebody to overstate problems in the NHS. She was challenged by counsel to the Mid-Staffordshire inquiry about her view that the first report into the hospital had used unnecessarily graphic language, saying: "If wards are filthy it should be said they were filthy. But I don't think we need to go into every spot of blood and every scrap of faeces, and every spit of sputum." So she is not one to overdramatise problems. Yet she found that still she could not speak freely but was "leaned on" to "tone down" what she was saying about NHS organisations.

An awareness that the message sent to the public needs to be carefully managed and controlled wherever possible has penetrated the innermost workings of the NHS. Take a look at the national requirements for reporting of serious incidents.* It includes a list of the types of incidents that must be reported, including, for example, wrong-site surgery. Fair enough. It includes events that lead to

---

* National Framework for Reporting and Learning from Serious Incidents Requiring Investigation, NHS Gateway Ref: 13733.

avoidable death. Again, very sensible. And it includes events that might lead to adverse media coverage. What?

This is a system that purports to help clinicians and managers learn from each other's mistakes. Operating on the wrong part of a patient is definitely a mistake. So is killing the patient. But according to what sort of values does encountering "adverse media coverage" count as a mistake? Certainly not any clinical standards, nor indeed any standards of common sense. The British media's ability to pillory the praiseworthy is something for which we are known around the globe. If I read an airline safety manual which said defects had to be reported if they might lead to "adverse media coverage" I would avoid getting on their planes.

It is there because the whole system is built to avoid surprises. That way, the secretaries and ministers of state can continue to calmly reassure the public that all is well. They behave like the captain of a liner with a hole in its hull who wanders the saloons assuring the passengers that everything is under control while down below decks everyone works furiously to patch the leaks. The last thing they want is some oil-smeared engineer bursting in yelling that it is all getting a bit difficult.

Let's go back to 3 June 2009. That was the day that Ben Bradshaw was assuring his colleagues in the House of Commons that the problems at Mid-Staffordshire were unique and that "no other trusts gave rise to similar concerns".

Anyone who had looked the data on NHS mortality that day – the same data that had given rise to the concerns at Mid-Staffordshire – would have noticed one hospital with a noticeably higher mortality rate than the rest. Basildon Hospital's mortality rate was far outside expected levels, more than 30 per cent above the expected rate for its patients and higher than Mid-Staffordshire's had been at its highest point. At that same moment, the regulator was forming its soon-to-be-published view that Basildon Hospital scored 13/14 for safety and was overall a "good" hospital. Four months later, this opinion would be reversed and Basildon Hospital would be in the headlines for failing to deliver a safe service.

The big lie matters because if we keep on pretending that we already know how to tell the difference between a good hospital and a bad hospital when, in truth, we don't, we will fail to do what is necessary to fix the problem.

CHAPTER 8

Sitting in judgement

The public inquiry into Mid-Staffordshire hospital's NHS Foundation Trust took place in the offices of Stafford borough council – a red-brick, low-rise office block at the end of the main street with a branch of the Royal Bank of Scotland and a shop selling discount white goods on the ground floor. Public inquiries are courts of law but they usually take place in municipal buildings requisitioned for the purpose. The inquiry has been given space on the fourth floor of the office building. A large function room with neutral fittings and strip lighting has been arranged with rows of desks facing the back of the room where Robert Francis QC, leading the inquiry, sits on a raised stage. His desk faces back at the rows of lawyers, reporters and interested members of the public. Unlike a normal court there is no dock. No one is on trial here. Or rather, everyone is. Everyone is here to account for themselves before a judge. We are here to apportion blame. This is the NHS on trial.

To his right, a desk has been arranged facing across the room at an angle. This is the witness stand. A cast list of over 150 people from ministers of state, the chief executive of the NHS, through all the ranks of regulators and managers, the doctors and the patients, all have sat here and given their version of events.

Everyone has been sorry for what has happened. And everyone has been able to put forward a good reason why they cannot be held responsible. The reasons are familiar. "I didn't know" remains the top favourite, usually with the supplementary: "There were not the resources available to uncover what was happening."

"I was doing what I was told" is in the top five. And then there is: "It was bad, but I was the one making things better."

This was the defence put forward by Martin Yeates, who was chief executive of the hospital during the period under investigation and who has subsequently suffered a breakdown which meant he could not testify in person. But in his statement to the inquiry the sense of outrage and the injustice he has suffered is palpable. He does not dispute that the hospital failed to look after patients as they should have. But it was the actions of others – the resources allocated to the hospital, the poor practices that had been allowed to develop before his arrival – that were to blame. The steps he was taking were going to fix the problem. It just had not quite happened at the point when the regulator decided to intervene.

I have been asked to give testimony. It is not something I have done before. I stand and swear to tell the "truth, the whole truth and nothing but the truth".

Brian Jarman has already given his testimony. He has explained how he developed his approach to mortality measurement, the way in which the figures were published by Dr Foster from 2001 onwards, and how, in 2007, they clearly showed that Mid-Staffordshire had a higher than expected mortality rate. These are the figures that should have alerted the hospital and others that something was badly wrong.

I am here to say a bit more about what had happened after we published the figures and to try to shed some light on why the figures had not acted as a warning sign to the hospital. It is a good question. The high mortality rates were the thing that finally pushed the regulator into an investigation. Why had the hospital itself not reacted in the same way?

It seems remarkable that at a time when patients were protesting about the care at the hospital, a study showing that many more patients were dying than you would expect failed to result in any problems being identified.

This was not through lack of action. Plenty of action was taken in response to the mortality figures, both by NHS managers in the hospital and those in other local NHS organisations. A group of academics were commissioned to investigate. They came up with methodological reasons why the statistical approach was unreliable. A group of data recording experts were hired who came back saying the problem was to do with the way data was being recorded. Public health doctors were asked their opinion and they came up with evidence that appeared to contradict the findings.

As it turned out, the academic doubts about methodology were misplaced, the problems with data accuracy were overstated and the evidence that seemed to contradict the findings only seemed to.

The questioning by the inquiry showed an understandable frustration at this situation. Why hadn't more been done to persuade the hospital to interpret the figures correctly? Why wasn't there greater consensus about what they meant?

In the time between the events at Mid-Staffordshire being under investigation and the inquiry taking place, the Department of Health took steps to address this. A group of experts was convened to discuss how hospitals should respond to data indicating high mortality rates. And the conclusion? The conclusion was that it should act as a prompt to further questions.

But isn't that exactly what the problem was in the first place? That instead of acting on the data the hospital simply asked more and more questions. At what point do they stop asking questions and come to a view on what is happening? Surely it could not be that hard to work out, from all the information that the management had, that there was a major problem.

To understand this it helps first to understand a bit about how people attempt to judge the quality of a health service.

A common approach is to break the problem into three parts and look at what are called in the jargon safety, effectiveness and experience. Safety means that the process of being treated did not actually harm you. It is the minimum you might expect. Effectiveness means that your treatment helped alleviate or cure your condition. Experience means you were treated decently by the people looking after you – that you were not ignored, or left waiting or made anxious because you did not know what was happening.

The lines between these different aspects of quality are not always obvious and can blur into one another. For example, a failure to wash hands which resulted in an infection would be a safety failing. But failure to operate in a timely fashion on a patient who then dies, in most cases, would not. It would be regarded as a failure to provide effective treatment. Or if a course of palliative treatment designed to reduce a patient's discomfort causes them a high level of anxiety it would be regarded as a poor experience rather than an ineffective course of treatment.

This is not a bad way to understand quality in healthcare. But there is another, rather different way of coming at the question, which looks at the different types of information you might use to determine how well a health service was doing.

The best answer put forward to this question came from the person who first started thinking about the problem. Avedis Donabedian was a remarkable man. He was born in Beirut in 1919 to Armenian parents and educated by Quakers in Ramallah before ending up in the US where, in addition to writing poetry, he became the first academic to start thinking seriously about how we tell how good a health service is.

Perhaps his best-known contribution to the debate was to suggest three different ways to answer the question. The first way, which he called "structure", was to ask if you had the sort of things you would expect to see in a good service. How many doctors have you got, how many hospital beds, how many health clinics, etc.? The good thing about this approach is that the things you are trying to count are relatively easy to count and the numbers will be fairly reliable. It is a good start since, plainly, if you have not got all these things, you probably do not have much of a health service. On the other hand, just because you have got all the kit, it does not mean it is all working the way it should.

The second way, he proposed, was to look at what these people did with all this stuff. This approach he called "process". The idea here is to describe what you think a good health service should do and then see if that is what is happening. Take polio vaccination, for example. The "structure" question is: do you have clinics with doctors who have access to the necessary vaccines? If not, you probably do not have much of a vaccination service. The "process" question is: how many people got vaccinated? It is all well and good having clinics and doctors but if they are not doing what they are supposed to, it helps no one.

There remains a school of thought which strongly advocates this as the best way to measure a health service. It requires a good deal of form-filling and paperwork but, if everyone fills out the forms correctly, you do get a clear answer. A high vaccination rate is, probably, a useful achievement. The data is not hard to interpret. If too few people were vaccinated it is not hard to know where to start to fix the problem.

The difficulty with this approach is that health processes are complicated. The process of making a vaccination programme work is not simply captured by knowing whether or not people were vaccinated. You would need to know, among many other things, that the vaccines were transported correctly and stored in the right way, that they were administered in the right doses and at the right time, that the people needing vaccination were correctly identified and so on. If any part of this process fails, the whole system fails.

In many areas of life, safety and quality are defined in terms of processes. If you are flying an aeroplane or running a nuclear power plant there are very long and extremely detailed manuals setting out the correct procedures for every activity. Quality control can then be done by auditing whether the specified procedures have been followed.

This approach is also used in healthcare. It is helpful. Clear rules about things as simple as how often and how you wash your hands have done wonders in reducing infection. But this solution on its own is not sufficient. The reason is simply that the scale of the data required to audit whole healthcare systems is unfeasibly large. To audit all the processes across a healthcare system for all the standards set for those activities would require box ticking on a gargantuan scale. The growing use of electronic patient records and clinical audit means that more and more of this data is being collected. But then there is the huge task of interpreting it all. And however much data you have, no amount of auditing processes would ever fully capture the complexity of delivering healthcare.

The third approach put forward by Donabedian was to look at what actually happens to the health of the patients. This is called looking at the "outcomes". To continue the vaccination example, the "outcome" question is: "How many people got polio?" Instead of trying to measure every aspect of the process you measure what matters most – whether or not it worked.

Most people would agree that measuring the outcome is, at least in theory, the most important way to measure the quality of a health service. It is hard to argue otherwise. After all, no amount of structure or process is worth a dime if in the end the outcomes are terrible. Also, measuring outcomes is a lot more cost-effective as you do not have to gather vast amounts of data about every step in the process.

The division into structure, process and outcome can be applied to any aspect of healthcare. For example, the outcome for safety is not whether hygiene standards were followed but whether or not the patient became infected. The outcome for experience is what the patients said they felt about the way they were treated, not what the hospital did.

The idea of moving towards measuring healthcare in terms of outcomes has been enthusiastically promoted as a central part of reforming the NHS by both Labour and the Conservatives over the past 15 years. It was a central plank of Andrew Lansley's case for reform. He argued that far too much NHS time was wasted collecting process data against government targets which often meant nothing. He worried that hospitals could often comply with these targets while failing to deliver the intended objective.

This was one of the issues that came up during the Mid-Staffordshire inquiry. During the questioning, I was shown tables of data used by the management of the trust to track performance. There was nothing particularly wrong with the information they were looking at, but it mainly included process measures, such as how long patients had waited to get into hospital, how long to be treated when they were there, how long to get discharged again. There was one outcome metric, which was whether patients became infected during their stay in hospital. The trust did well on nearly all the metrics. Except this one.

By having one or two bits of information that related to the outcomes of care, the hospital management were able to argue that they were looking at quality. By mixing these up with a lot of information about details of the process – such as how long the patient waited – they were able to tell themselves that overall, on balance, they were doing well. It obscured the fact that, on the things that measured the quality of their care they were not doing well and that the things they did well on did not relate to quality.

The NHS is now moving towards adopting outcomes as the measure of quality, but this change conflicts with the culture of an organisation that is intolerant of surprises and values managerial control. Compared to processes, outcomes are far less amenable to management by diktat and measurement of them far more challenging.

You might imagine that measuring the outcome would be easy – after all the one thing you would expect a health service to know is how healthy its patients are. But the problem is that you are not simply trying to measure the health of your patients and see whether or not they get better. Even if I knew exactly how healthy all my patients were that would not tell me anything about how good my health service is. They might all just be unusually healthy people.

To know how good healthcare is you have to assess the extent to which it has changed the health of patients. In other words I need to know not just how healthy my patients are, I also have to be able to compare this with how healthy they would have been if they had not been treated by me. This is challenging. How do you tell how healthy people would have been in circumstances that never took place?

Just how hard this is can be seen from attempts that have been made to look at patient records and assess whether the outcome would have been better if the care provided had been different. One approach is to review deaths and try to determine if any of them were avoidable. The results show how difficult this is to judge. In one widely cited study of deaths in hospitals the conclusion was that about 6 per cent of the deaths were certainly or probably avoidable. But 22.7 per cent of deaths were "possibly" avoidable.*

There is a huge number of scenarios in that 22.7 per cent. Maybe if the patient had had better hydration, or had someone help them eat that evening, it might have made them stronger and enabled them to recover and survive. Maybe the patient's observations were not checked when they should have been shortly before the patient died. Perhaps if they had been it would have indicated deterioration and prompted a response that might have saved the patient. But then maybe it would not have. Who can say? The list of things that *might* have made a difference is very long indeed. And it is rare that

---

* R Hayward, T Hoffer, Estimating hospital deaths due to medical error: preventability is in the eye of the reviewer. JAMA, vol. 286, no. 4, 2001.

a specific event can be said to have definitely caused the death of a patient.

Assessing whether a certain event has or has not contributed to the death of a patient becomes harder the closer you are to that event. When Mid-Staffordshire Hospital was trying to understand why it had such a high mortality rate, it formed a group of clinicians to look into the issue. They decided to review the case notes of 35 patients who had died in the hospital to see if they could find anything that might have been done differently. Their conclusion was that death was entirely "predictable" in 34 of the 35 cases – only one death was unexpected. Furthermore, in only five of the cases could they find any fault with the care provided.*

If you regard a particular person's death as predictable it can make you behave in strange ways. June Chell was one of the people who came forward to the original Mid-Staffordshire inquiry to talk about her experiences. She explained how her husband was admitted to hospital as an emergency and died. During his stay he was assaulted by another patient on the ward who put his hands round his neck and tried to strangle him. Her husband never spoke again, from that night until the morning he died.

---

* Investigation into Mid-Staffordshire NHS Foundation Trust, Healthcare Commission, March 2009.

She recounts a great many indignities suffered during that period but one in particular is relevant here. After her husband's death her son went to collect the death certificate from the hospital. While there, he asked the head nurse about the assault. The nurse replied: "It made no difference."

Apart from the fact that, as June Chell put it, "I don't know how she could say that to someone who had just lost his dad," it is concerning that someone might so easily judge an event of this sort to have "made no difference". If you think it is entirely "predictable" that someone is going to die, it might affect how you treat them.

When the Healthcare Commission started to investigate the hospital, it decided to carry out a quick check of the work of the mortality group. It selected eight sets of patient notes that had been reviewed by the group and repeated the exercise. The eight cases included the one where the hospital had said the death was not expected and seven where the death was regarded as "predictable". The view of the regulator was rather different. Their experts thought that in only two of the eight cases was death expected, and there were concerns about the way all the other patients had been handled.

Reviewing case notes is an important part of any good system of quality control (or clinical governance, as it is called) in hospital. But when opinions about what is concerning and what is predictable can diverge so widely it is unwise to put too much reliance on this type of process as an assurance that nothing is going wrong. Indeed, it is exactly in the sort of hospital where things are going wrong that you might expect to find less rigour in the case note reviews.

So is there, perhaps, a more objective way of coming at the question of avoidable deaths? One approach involves not looking at individual patients but looking at a large numbers of patients. By seeing if, on average, patients being treated differently are experiencing different outcomes, it may be possible to start to judge which aspects of health-care are producing good outcomes and which are not.

This is the approach taken by Professor Sir Brian Jarman. Brian Jarman is partly an epidemiologist. Epidemi-ologists are doctors who use statistics to study the way in which illness occurs in populations and to understand what is causing those illnesses. Despite the fact that this is what he is most famous for, Professor Jarman does not regard himself first and foremost as an epidemiologist. Unlike many of his colleagues, he has also been, throughout his career, a practising doctor – a GP in central London. This has given him a rather different perspective. It has enabled him to combine the viewpoint of someone who looks at healthcare up close in the surgery, day by day, patient by patient, with the mile-high view provided by health statistics.

Traditionally epidemiologists use statistics to understand what causes illness in a population. They study questions such as how infectious diseases spread through a country or how lifestyle decisions like smoking or healthy eating affect our health. Professor Jarman chose to do something rather different. He used the same data to try to understand the extent to which our hospitals and doctors are making people healthier. He turned the data back on the system and started to question the degree to which healthcare organisations really do make people better.

Professor Jarman's approach to analysis of hospital mortality rates is now used in many countries around the world but were first published here in the UK through the Dr Foster Hospital Guide as an independent assessment of quality of hospital care.

It is an approach that is designed to directly address the question that we find so difficult to answer – who is providing good healthcare and who is not? Unlike many of the questions epidemiologists address, this one is distinctly uncomfortable. You are guaranteed to have somebody who does not like your answer.

If you do not like the answer, it is easy to cast doubt on the finding. "How do you really know that my patients would not have died if something else had happened?" The statistics tell us that a very similar group of patients treated elsewhere and in a different manner survived better. But it is never possible to say for sure that the actual patients treated by a particular doctor in a particular location would have fared any better or worse in different circumstances. It may be that the apparent differences are caused by influences that we do not understand or which are not properly recorded in the data. There are lots of statistical techniques to iron out these differences and adjust for them, but if someone does not believe the result reflects anything they did, there is rarely any way of proving the point either way.

In this regard it is very different from measuring processes. If you can show patients did not receive the vaccination, there is no disputing the facts. If you show that higher numbers of people than expected contracted polio, you will rarely be able to say for certain why that occurred.

In scientific studies, when trying to understand whether a particular medicine or treatment works, randomised trials are used. In a randomised trial, the patients who receive the new medicine are selected at random and are compared to another set of patients also selected at random from the same population. Because both groups are selected randomly, it is fair to assume that there will be no systematic differences between them aside from the treatment they receive. That is why it is generally safe to conclude that any differences are due to the difference in the medicines taken.

But if you are comparing the patients treated by one doctor or one hospital with the patients treated by another we are certainly not comparing two randomly selected groups of patients. They will probably live in different areas and the fact that a group of patients all go to the same place for treatment may well reflect something else in common between them.

I have spent many hours presenting information to hospital managers about various analyses that purport to show how their outcomes compare. The immediate response to figures showing a good outcome is usually a smile followed by an enthusiastic "That's interesting." When the outcome is poor the response is almost always to suggest, first, that it would be unsafe to place any great reliance on the results since there are known to be problems with the accuracy of the data (this is a safe bet as there is no data set yet created that is perfectly accurate). The next response is to observe that in this part of the country, patients are noticeably sicker than similar patients in other parts of the country.

It is almost impossible to discuss these data without worries about blame starting to obscure the issues. I remember an animated discussion with a doctor at one hospital who had been sent data showing that a high number of patients with acute renal failure admitted to the hospital had died. She responded by calling up details of some of the patients included in the analysis. The first was someone who had arrived at the hospital with renal failure, had been successfully treated with antibiotics, but who had then contracted pneumonia on the ward and died. Her complaint was that it was unfair to describe this as a death following admission with renal failure since this implied she, the renal physician, was to blame. The patient might have died but if it was the result of pneumonia then that was not her fault. In the debate about blame, the fact patients were dying in the hospital from avoidable causes rather got lost.

This is why people are much more comfortable with process measures. With a process measure it is, on the whole, easy to identify the cause, easy to assign responsibility, easy to put in place measures that appear to remedy the problem. With outcome measures it all becomes a great deal more complicated.

In 2010, the Department of Health published an Outcomes Framework for the English NHS that identifies key aspects of care that will be measured, including stopping people from dying prematurely, ensuring people recover quickly from periods of illness, making life better for people with long-term conditions and improving people's experience of care.

This is an important step in the right direction. But changing from an organisation that runs on tightly managed process targets to one that aims to improve outcomes is proving to be a gradual process. The operating framework for the NHS in 2012 was not so very different from the framework within which Mid-Staffordshire was operating in 2008. The plan for 2013 does look very different with the standards against which the NHS says it will measure itself dominated by outcome measures. But there is ambivalence about how this will affect the way the NHS operates. David Nicholson, in an interview with the Health Service Journal, made the following observation about the changes taking place: "There were some strengths to the way in which we operated in the past – the clarity, the direction – the unequivocal, one definition of success. All that is really important."[*]

An unequivocal single definition of success is what the NHS machine is built to work with. It is how the process measures and targets operate. They are unambiguous. Either the box has a tick or it does not. These are the things that bureaucracy knows how to do well. To change

---

[*] Nicholson will not give away his "grip". Health Service Journal, 17 Jan. 2013

to a world in which outcomes really are assessed will be a challenge. It will require a wholly different way of operating. It will be like watching a dolphin learning to walk.

That is not intended as a slur on NHS bureaucracy. It is merely a reflection of how bureaucracies like to work. Working with outcome measures is something that any good bureaucracy will find much more challenging than dealing with processes. But it is essential to find a way of doing it. In our favour is the fact that NHS bureaucracy is an unusually competent bureaucracy with a great many motivated and smart people working for it. It is endlessly denigrated but, in truth, comprises a competent and skilled group of people with some very effective ways of working. If any bureaucracy is going to find a way of working with outcomes, I would back the NHS.

But that does not alter the fact that it has a way of working that does not sit easily with the need to move towards running a health service on the basis of the outcomes it achieves. To do that, it is going to have to learn some new tricks. If the NHS treats outcomes like a new set of performance targets, much effort will go into doing whatever is necessary to get the numbers to look right, even if the reality is rather different. Working with outcomes is going to require a whole new approach to understanding how well organisations are doing at looking after their patients.

That is the real reason why the problems at Mid-Staffordshire did not get identified from the data. It was because the NHS was looking at the wrong data. And the reason the NHS was looking at the wrong data was because it does not know how to interpret and act on the right data.

Back at the Mid-Staffordshire inquiry, as Robert Francis listens to all the evidence in front of him, he is trying to work out what has gone wrong. Who did the wrong thing, who did the right thing, where did things work as they should have done, where did the system break down? He is not using a set of performance metrics to try to do this, he is listening to a series of conflicting accounts, trying to form a coherent picture of what happened so he can then form a judgement. It is exactly the sort of process that is needed to untangle complex information and make sense of it. It requires the sorts of skills you would need to try to run the NHS on outcomes. Unfortunately it is a set of skills and behaviours that are still a world away from the NHS.

CHAPTER 9

Other worlds

I am writing this in the week before the 2012 US election. Elections are fascinating, if you are interested in data and the way information is used. Opinion polls plays two very different roles in an election. They are there primarily to help the different participants – the media, the campaign managers, the bookies laying odds – to understand what voters are thinking so they can plan accordingly. But they do not just describe events, they also affect them. They become part of the information voters use to decide what they think and what they plan to do. Knowing that one candidate is miles ahead in the polls makes a difference to how people behave. It may, for example, have an influence on whether or not you choose to get out of bed early and walk through the rain to the polling station.

Polling is a complex science. Polls are what would be called in healthcare an indicator. They try to measure what is going on out there in the real world. They are not unlike some of the metrics used to try to understand what is happening to the health of patients. They can never be perfect but they are useful nonetheless. And like healthcare metrics, the answer you get depends to a significant degree on how you put the information together.

The results of a poll are not like the results of an election. They are a statistical artefact and there is as much art as science to how you put them together. The result you get from a poll depends on where and how you select the people to take part and, even more, on how you choose to model the results. To turn the raw data of people's answers into a opinion poll result you have to adjust the data to take account of all sorts of unknown influences. For example, you make assumptions about how well one person's opinions represent the views of others or how well their answers reflect how they will actually behave. Just because someone tells a pollster they definitely intend to vote for Obama does not mean that they will actually bother to get to a polling station and vote.

This leaves a fair amount of room for apparently identical polls to produce very different results. In the week running up to the election, most polling organisations were showing the two candidates, Obama and Romney, even on 49 per cent each. But a poll from Gallup showed Romney a clear 4 points ahead of Obama at 50 per cent to 46 per cent. This is no surprise – Gallup polls have consistently shown Romney in the lead. So has another organisation called Rasmussen. It is run by a group of Republicans and the polls are widely used in Republican campaign litera- ture. Equally, there are a number of "left-leaning" polls. For example Ipsos/Reuters has consistently produced results that put Obama in the lead. All these organisations are trying to measure the same thing. But they are getting very different results.

It is no great surprise that different methodologies can produce results favouring one candidate or the other. But this does not matter. It does not render the information useless. Because the information is not used to select the president. The president is not chosen on the basis of an opinion poll, the president is chosen through an election.

The difference is important. An election is not an attempt to measure anything. It is not an attempt to assess the views of the population. There are many more accurate ways to do that. An election is an event. It is a method of selecting people to govern. It is a way of appointing leaders who are not wholly intolerable to the rest of us. We use them because, in the main, they do that reasonably well and people accept the results. They are not perfect but they are a legitimate way of discriminating between acceptable and unacceptable politicians.

Opinion polls are useful because they help us understand elections. The people who use opinion poll data to make decisions about campaigns are very skilled at it. They know how to work with imperfect data and piece information together to get a real understanding of what it is telling them about what is happening out there in the real world. One thing they do not do, however, is start to think that the poll results are more important than elections or what is happening out there in the real world.

It is the same in other walks of life. Take finance. It is a world in which data is used continuously by analysts and commentators to understand what is happening to companies and share prices. The aim of the whole exercise is to discriminate between well-managed, profitable, growing companies and poorly managed, loss-making businesses. Doing this involves using tons of data. There are regulators who set down rules about what data must be made available by companies. Other people collect data about markets and trends and sales volumes and profit margins. Analysts sift through the numbers and rank companies, develop different approaches to interpreting the information, build models that predict which companies are succeeding and which are not.

But how a company performs on an analyst's score card is not what matters. The information is there to inform the decisions of shareholders who decide whether to invest in a company or sell it, who decide whether to vote to keep the directors at the Annual General Meeting or replace them.

In both these worlds there is a clear difference between information, on the one hand, and real decisions and judgements on the other. No amount of data analysis in the world can susbstitute for the judgements made by investors. No amount of opinion poll data can ever substitute for the judgement of the people expressed at an election. Data exists to try to understand what is happening out in the real world. It is there to help people make judgements.

This is not how data is used in the NHS. In the NHS, instead of using data to understand what is happening in the real world, the data instead becomes a substitute for it.

In the world of NHS performance management, performance scorecards are not like analyst's reports – a view of the world that may help inform a judgement. They *are* the judgement. The way bureaucracy works is to take a problem or an objective and turn it into a series of metrics and processes which can be implemented and audited so that all the boxes are ticked and all the forms filed. That is what good bureaucracies do with tremendous efficiency. However, once the problem has been reduced to a series of numbers, getting the numbers right, the processes complete and the boxes ticked becomes the objective, regardless of how well it corresponds to the original objective.

The NHS Outcomes Framework is a fine document which sets out a sensible set of measures that aim to describe what a good healthcare system would look like. It is a very useful document. The only problem is that it does not actually describe good healthcare. It is an approximation for convenience. It is exactly the sort of approximation that should be in use – just so long as we remember that it is an approximation, not the real thing.

The affliction that struck the NHS and made it unable to see what was happening in Mid-Staffordshire was not simply caused by the fact that people were looking at the wrong numbers – processes instead of outcomes. It was also, to a significant degree, the inevitable consequence of a system that all too readily substitutes a scorecard for any form of real judgement.

This is not an argument against using data. Without data about quality in healthcare we are lost. But it is an argument against using data without judgement. It is an argument against the bureaucratic approach to data.

Let us go back, for a minute, to the three reports delivered to Lord Darzi in 2008 from Joint Commission International, The Institute for Healthcare Improvement and the Rand Corporation.

All three organisations were asked to examine the systems for ensuring healthcare quality in England and comment on how they could be improved. The reports, which came to remarkably similar conclusions, were not published by the Department of Health and only came to light after a freedom of information request by a thinktank, the Policy Exchange, after a tip-off from Brian Jarman.

One of the most interesting observations made by two of the reports noted that the constant efforts to reform the NHS have been one of the biggest obstacles to improvement. As the Institute for Healthcare Improvement put it, if all the money that had been spent on redundancies caused by reorganisation had instead been put into improvement it might have made quite a difference. We can only guess what they would make of the latest extravaganza of desk-shifting under a confetti cloud of P45s.

But the thing that came through most strongly in all three reports was the issue of culture in the NHS – the fact that the management of healthcare organisations "looked up, not out". Imagine the NHS as a pyramid of power in which the secretary of state at the top has most power, senior managers are next in line for power, followed by junior managers. Finally, at the bottom of the pyramid, you have the patients, with little or no power. The observation of all three organisations was that NHS employees looked to where the power was. The thing that loomed largest in their thinking was whatever their superiors were demanding. The demands of patients and the wider world outside were very much in second place.

They all called for a change in culture – although how this was to be achieved no one was able to say in any great detail.

For clues to how this might be possible, it helps to look at how things operate in some of those other worlds – the worlds of politics, business, or even law. What stops these worlds from becoming inward-looking bureaucracies? What, if anything, connects them to the real world?

The first thing to note is that, in these worlds, the way in which judgements are made has a high degree of public acceptance and legitimacy. They may not be perfect but they are recognised as, on the whole, fair. In politics, elections are influenced by many things and at times the results can look questionable, but on the whole we accept that elections are probably the best means we have to discriminate between people who should be allowed to take charge and people who should not.

Similarly, in business, shareholders make judgements about the management of companies. These judgements will often be flawed, poorly informed or just wrong. But, on the whole, they have proved an effective way of telling the difference between a good business and a bad one. We broadly accept the judgements of investors as a legitimate means of appointing directors to companies and distributing investment funds.

In the same way, the courts are our mechanism for discriminating between people who have broken the law and those who have not. It is not a perfect system. We know there is a difference between being innocent in the eyes of God and being found innocent by a court. But the two are sufficiently close that the latter is seen as an acceptable approximation of the former.

The NHS does not have an equivalent. The organisations and individuals tasked with assessing the quality of healthcare organisations lack the same degree of legitimacy. Getting a green light from the regulator is not a credible indication that an organisation is providing high-quality healthcare, nor is getting an OK from your local NHS commissioning organisation, nor is performing well on the NHS performance framework.

There is a troubling void where there ought to be people making judgements. And where they do exist, on the whole, instead of using data to inform judgements, data is used as a substitute for making judgements.

Too often, real judgement is replaced with formulaic exercises. The way in which the CQC registered healthcare organisations was claimed to be an exercise in which a wide range of information sources were used to check that organisations were qualified to provide health services. An alternative view of what was going on was given by the whistle-blower Amanda Pollard, who contacted the Mid-Staffordshire inquiry to say that she felt the description that had been given of this process was inaccurate. She had been one of the people tasked with registering organisations and stated that it had become nothing more than a paper-processing exercise. As long as all the boxes were ticked on the relevant forms, the organisation got its registration. No one was exercising any real judgement.

The appraisal of doctors is another moment where, in theory, a degree of judgement is applied. Doctors must be appraised each year by their NHS employer and, every five years, the appraisal will include a review of whether they are fit to continue to practise. The description of the process as set out in the official manuals requires the doctor to produce a wide range of information about their activity and evidence that they are performing well. But the reality, according to many, is that, as long as there is a piece of paper in the right file with the right type of information on it, everybody is happy. The extent to which this information can truly be said to have been reviewed and used to make a judgement about the strengths and weaknesses of that particular doctor is questionable if not completely absent.

The NHS has in the past been very clear about the way in which it works and judgement is very much given a back seat. Take for example, the 2012 Performance Framework for the NHS. It sets out in clear terms the principles for assessing performance of NHS organisation.* It includes a commitment to be transparent by having "clear and predetermined performance measures" as well as "a uniform approach across England, at different levels of the system and across different types of providers".

By limiting itself to "pre-agreed" measures of performance and by restricting itself to using a "uniform approach", the whole system has, from the outset, limited its ability to make any real judgements.

If you are really trying to judge how well an NHS organisation is doing you want every piece of information you can get your hands on and you want to try every approach to interpreting it. You would not limit yourself to a "uniform approach" using "pre-agreed" measures.

---

* The NHS Performance Framework: Implementation Guidance 2012/13.

The NHS does this because it is thought to be a fairer way of operating. If you are going to judge someone, you first have to tell them how you are going to score the test. That's the fair way, even if it does not work very well. The NHS documents make clear that these programmes of work are not intended to preclude other local organisations from making their own judgements. But when everybody operates in this way, you are left with a world in which no one is making any judgements.

Judgement is unpopular in the NHS because it is chaotic and messy. Elections, court cases, investment decisions are unpredictable and often cause upset. That is how things are in the real world. For a bureaucracy such unpredictability creates confusion and that is the worst of all evils. People are unsure where they stand. They might be forced to make judgements of their own.

Combine this outlook with a political culture that demands no unpleasant surprises, and it is impressive that so many people in the NHS manage to focus on more than their latest performance spreadsheet.

One thing that makes it particularly hard for the NHS to base itself on judgement is the lack of informed debate. Where there should be discussion there is silence. Compare what happens in the worlds of politics, law and business. They all thrive on debate and conflicting opinions. Companies are not assessed on a set of "pre-agreed" measures. They are constantly assessed and re-assessed using different approaches that produce quite different viewpoints. One analysis will indicate a company is doing much better than its peers, another will suggest it is heading for trouble.

This is fantastically useful to people who have to make judgements as it tests out the different possible interpretations of the data. Furthermore, if you ever find that everyone is agreeing then it is a pretty telling sign.

Politics works in exactly the same way. The media provides a forum in which differing accounts of candidates' strengths can be played out to help inform judgements. A court is a very formalised version of exactly the same process. It is a structured arena in which conflicting opinions can be played out and tested.

The debate about what is good or poor in the NHS is conducted through a rather sterile internal process that takes place in meeting rooms where people decide what the "pre-agreed" measures of performance are going to be. True, there is an entirely separate, rather more vigorous, parallel public debate in the press. But this is, in comparison, often poorly informed and driven by anecdote. Consequently, those on the inside tend to regard it as ignorant, intrusive and a distraction from the proper work of the health service.

For the NHS to change its culture to become less inward-looking is an enormous challenge. To do that it would need to do two things. It would need to become much more skilled in making judgements about quality. One of the main benefits of this would be the ability to recognise success much more than it does.

The three US reports into how quality was managed in the NHS made the point that there were few incentives for managers in the NHS to aim high. They are punished for failing to meet targets, but they are not rewarded for excelling in anything. An NHS skilled in judging quality would have much greater freedom to acknowledge where people are doing amazing things that never get captured on the official performance figures.

The other thing it could do would be to try to encourage more diverse opinions on what is working and what is not working. The NHS has traditionally been shy of encouraging outside comment and nervous about the results. But that is starting to change. Transparency has been another theme of reform in the NHS for the past 10 years. The idea is that the NHS will be very open about the information it holds and allow other organisations to look at this data and make their own judgements about how well things are working.

Dr Foster was the first real attempt to bring an independent assessment of what was good and bad about NHS organisations. Across much of the NHS it was wholly unwelcome and regarded as thoroughly illegitimate and unfair.

The complaint was that the way we judged hospitals was not "pre-agreed", it was not something they understood. Another complaint was that it was confusing to the public to have people saying something that does not agree with official views of NHS organisations. And there were complaints that what we were doing was fundamentally undemocractic. The elected government had a mandate from the people to determine what the NHS should aim to do. It was not down to anyone else to start trying to interfere with that process.

The medical professions were equally ambivalent. If the NHS does not take kindly to external comments on its performance, doctors can be even more frosty. When Dr Foster first published mortality rates for heart surgery, the reaction of some surgeons was unprintable. It was not because they were against transparency. Under the leadership of Bruce Keogh, now Medical Director of the NHS, they led the way in publishing information about their outcomes. They were enthusiastic about having information about the success or otherwise of their treatment. Despite this, many of them remained profoundly uncomfortable with the idea that people they considered less qualified to speak might comment on their performance.

After leaving university I worked for a while at the Consumers' Association, which published Which? magazine. One of the bits of folklore about the history of Which? magazine was the extent to which the manufacturers of fridges and kettles responded with legal threats when it was first proposed that Which? intended to publish ratings of their products. They did not believe it was possible that anyone could accurately capture the sophisticated and subtle differences between one fridge and another through crude rating mechanisms and the results would be wholly misleading.

They pointed out that, however scientifically you measure the different aspects of a kettle, putting it together into an overall assessment will inevitably be arbitrary. That is true. But making these sorts of arbitrations is exactly the aim of the process.

A similar process is starting to take place now in healthcare. The patient group Macmillan Cancer Support recently published an assessment of cancer services in which it found that Harrogate Hospital had the best cancer care in the country and Imperial College Hospital in London the worst. It was not a comprehensive assessment. It did not look at patient outcomes or safety. It looked only at measures of patient experience. The information used was not new. The surveys of patients on which it was based had been available for some time. What made it striking was the act of turning the data into an assessment of the quality of different services. The simple process of reviewing the figures and coming to a clear conclusion as to who was doing well and who was not was important.

It is important because it makes it harder to ignore the data. Using data on its own, it is easy to think your way out of the implications, to tell yourself that a change in the sample size would have altered the result or that the way the measures were calculated failed to take account of local differences. Too often, in hospitals that have poor survey results, the prevailing opinion is that the data is unreliable and the picture created is out of sync with experience.

By making a clear judgement, Macmillan publicly challenged such readings. That matters. Because if you can write off the data in your own mind and no one else is paying it much attention, nothing will happen. It is only when that thinking is challenged credibly that there is any likelihood that we can start to see the connections between data and the real world.

When Dr Foster started to publish ratings of hospitals in 2001, it was regarded as wicked by many in the NHS. It was felt to be an ambush. It was unfair because people had not been told in advance that hospitals might be rated in this fashion. There was very little understanding of the idea that looking at data anew – avoiding the pre-agreed way of viewing the world and coming up with a different perspective – is essential to properly understanding information. And it is vital if interpretation of data is not to loose its mooring to real-world events.

Many people felt that having differing opinions made their job impossible because they did not know which way to turn. In reality, the true risks lay in the opposite direction. The bigger risk is that having a very clear and fixed idea of what should be done makes it easy to ignore the evidence that these actions are failing to produce the desired result.

A common complaint about this sort of assessment is the notion that it is 'unscientific'. Science, after all, is not about entertaining conflicting opinions – it is about identifying the truth. This is to wholly misunderstand the process of science. Just like politics or business, science is a process of making judgements by sifting through reams of conflicting evidence. There is hardly a scientific theory on earth that does not still have someone out there willing to call it into question. That is the whole strength of the scientific establishment. It works because it provides a mechanism for claims and counter-claims to be tested and judgements made. Admittedly, the question of what constitutes good healthcare is never going to be amenable to the sort of definitive answer that can be reached on many questions in science. But that does not make it any less important to come to a judgement.

Encouraging conflicting opinions is important because the act of measuring an organisation inevitably corrupts it. There is no way round this. It does not mean we should stop doing it. But we need to recognise that the moment you start to measure an organisation in a particular way it starts to bend that organisation out of shape.

The intention of measuring a health service is to identify where things are working and fix them. But, in a world where often the metric has replaced judgement, it is inevitable that the pressure to perform against the data causes other things to happen as well.

People start to change the way they do things so that it *looks* as if the service has improved, even if it has not. So, for example, if you are being measured on how many patients are seen within four hours in A&E, you can either increase the number of patients seen within four hours. Or you can keep patients waiting longer on trolleys prior to allowing them into the A&E for assessment so that the clock starts ticking later. Or you can admit them into an "observation ward" within four hours and then you can take as long as you like to get round to treating them.

Another option is to simply change the way you record what you do so that the metrics improve even if the service remains the same. So, for example, hospital mortality rates are adjusted to take account of how ill patients are. By simply recording information about your patients which makes them appear sicker, it is possible to make your adjusted mortality rate come down.

If we are to have an NHS that is managed to produce good outcomes for patients, this needs to be addressed by being much more rigorous in ensuring that patient records are accurate. In business, the consequence of mis-recording your sales figures or your income is a charge of fraud and a long stretch in jail. In the NHS the consequence of mis-recording what happened to patients is often nothing at all. If we are going to have an NHS run on outcomes that will not do.

We also need to recognise that the susceptibility of these measures to flaws in the data is another reason why information of this sort must inform judgements, not become a substitute for them. The numbers need to be examined carefully, alternative interpretations of the data considered, and an assessment made.

To move away from a blame culture driven by a requirement to meet central targets and an aversion to surprises, we need to move towards a more open culture of frank assessment and skilled judgement. This does not mean a culture in which criticism is muted. It means the opposite. It means a culture in which there is an open discussion about what is good and what is bad about our health services. It means a culture in which criticism can be made without it being seen as an "attack" on the NHS. It means a culture in which patient complaints are treated with respect, not with fear and defensiveness.

It implies a culture in which there is debate and disagreement about the NHS. But – and this is the hope – it means a culture in which that argument is grounded in better informed efforts to understand what is happening to patients. It is one in which it is very hard for NHS organisations to lose track of the reality of what is happening in wards, waiting rooms and clinics. It is one in which the many and often conflicting voices of patients, the public and the world outside is louder than the voices of managers and ministers.

Both the current and the previous administrations have pursued policies of greater transparency and more open data. There has been considerable hope that this would lead to exactly this sort of culture of debate. It was hoped that "armchair auditors" would appear and that patient representative groups would start to use the data to challenge NHS organisations. In the event, there has been relatively little uptake of the information. But this is hardly surprising. It was rather optimistic to hope that citizens would take up the challenge of making sense of complex health statistics. The data is highly technical and the skills required to interpret it in short supply. But the goal remains the right one. And further steps to encourage more diverse opinion on NHS performance should be a goal of any administration that wants to make the NHS more outward looking.

The task of truly understanding where health services are working well and where they are not is a major undertaking. And it cannot be achieved without the help of each individual under the care of the NHS.

For this to work, we must all contribute. And the thing we need to contribute is not our taxes. The thing we need to contribute is information about ourselves.

Our understanding of what makes us sick and what makes us well is developing at an astonishing rate and in surprising directions. On one level, scientists are unravelling the human genome and learning how medicines and treatments that work for one person may be useless on another. At the other end of the spectrum, we are starting to understand just how complex the idea of "good health" really is – that the connection between good health (both physical and mental) and a good life (in terms of being happy and able to live as we would chose) is not straightforward. As more and more of us spend greater amounts of time alive but unwell, healthcare becomes not just about curing illness but equally about finding the best way to live with our physical and mental infirmities.

To be able to find the combination of care, support, treatment and medication that works for our particular circumstances means coming at the question in a way that lets us balance the therapeutic benefits of joining a social club and making friends against the therapeutic benefits of medicines and machinery. We need to understand not just whether one drug works better than another at reducing symptoms. We need to know in what circumstances and for what patients, that particular drug works. We need to begin to try to identify the combinations of factors make the most difference to people's lives.

The answers may surprise us. The thing that makes the patients in one area recover more quickly from illness or cope better with disability may be the precise combination of treatments they receive, it may be their genetic disposition or it may be something as simple as the respect with which the doctors and nurses speak to them.

To understand what is happening, we need to understand much better how the whole of the care system affects our lives. To do this, we need to do more than the sort of traditional medical research that tests whether particular treatments have an effect on the patient's illness. We need to start understanding much better how both social care and health services improve patients' overall wellbeing.

The ability to do this is now within our grasp because of the computerisation of health information. Today, in the UK, there are relatively few facts about your health that are not recorded somewhere on an electronic database. To some people that is a deeply troubling fact. For others, it opens up fantastic opportunities.

Despite the failure of the NHS national programme for IT to create a single NHS electronic record, it remains the case that every attendance at your GP practice is recorded on a database along with every prescription made out to you. Every attendance at hospital and every operation is recorded on the hospital administration system and most test result is recorded on laboratory systems. As we put this data together we come to know an astonishing amount about what is happening to us.

Healthcare researchers and pharmaceutical companies are starting to use what is called "real-world evidence". Instead of carrying out specially constructed tests in which patients are given a new compound and specific measures are taken of their symptoms, they are starting to use these sources of data to understand the full long-term impact of different courses of treatment.

We are beginning to patch together the data from different computer systems, or manage patient information on a single electronic record. We can then anonymise the data, pool it all together and start to unpick what it all means. Primary care records from GPs are being linked with hospital records, and pathology lab records, and social care records to understand the impact of the whole of healthcare on our lives. More and more, these records are being supplemented with the patient's own reports of their health status.

There are some who object to this whole endeavour on the grounds that it invades patients' privacy. They are right to raise the issue. Using data in this way creates risks of misuse or loss of information. It is entirely correct to insist on rigorous standards in the way in which information is used in order to protect the confidentiality of individuals. It is understandable to be concerned about – and object to – large amounts of data being in the hands of governments or powerful organisations without very full legal controls.

But calls for this to stop or demands that patients be allowed to withdraw their information are misplaced. The development of modern medicine through the last century was driven by scientific discovery. We need to put in place the ability to take an equally scientific approach to the development of 21st-century health and care services. Having the information on which to do this is the first requirement.

We are fortunate in the UK that a single National Health Service means we are in a better position than most countries to be able to do this. When the NHS was founded in 1948 it was about all of us pooling our financial resources to make sure we were all looked after. In the coming century it will be as much about us all pooling the information about our lives, to ensure that we know how to best look after each other.

This can be done in ways that protect patients' privacy and which at the same time open up opportunities of such enormous public benefit that it is inconceivable we will turn away from them. The difficulty that such proposals encounter, is that the benefits are often expressed as "public benefits" rather than benefits to the individual.

We accept that banks hold our financial records on centralised computers, in part because it seems obvious that it would not be feasible to run a bank in another way, but also because we benefit directly. The fact that it is possible to travel the world with a single piece of plastic and draw cash instantly in any city on the globe is a wonder of the modern age.

If we are to accept our medical records being held on computers, we need to be offered more than the ill-defined promises of future improvements in our health services. We need to see how it makes life better for us individually. It must be done in a way that puts more power into the hands of patients.

CHAPTER 10

A patient
with power

Breaks Cafe is in a parade of single-storey shop fronts along the A518 as it comes into Stafford town centre. A steady stream of cars and lorries rumbles past, stopping periodically for the lights. On one side is a Chinese takeaway, on the other an "Asian" takeaway. Opposite, an imposing brick and stone edifice was built at the start of the last century to house Stafford library and museum. The library was relocated in 1999 and the building is now being advertised for commercial rent as a potential nightclub. It is a good idea. It would nicely complement the Apollo cinema next door and the nearby Weatherspoons bar.

The cafe has one main room with four square wooden tables, each with four wooden chairs. A man is washing dishes in the small kitchen out the back. Signs on the wall advertise the options – Jam sponge and custard £2.20, Oatcake with hot berries and ice cream £2.50. "If u don't see what you fancy, please ask."

I arrive early to talk to Julie and she is still busy closing up so she brings me a cup of tea, a large slice of sponge cake and asks me to wait. I listen to Elvis singing "Fools rush in, where angels fear to tread" playing from the music system on the counter.

A man opposite me in a bomber jacket and jeans is eating a sandwich. We start talking about oatcakes. Oatcakes – oatmeal pancakes – are the local specialty of Staffordshire. Well, certain parts of Staffordshire, he explains. They are popular in Stoke, around the potteries areas and in Stafford. "But Cannock doesn't bother with them," he explains, referring to the town 10 miles away.

He tells me that two weeks ago the last of the traditional bakers closed down – sole traders working out of terraced houses and selling oatcakes across counters built into the front window. Now they are all manufactured by large bakeries, he says.

Julie finishes for the day and comes to sit with me. She is a small figure with a manner that is kind if wary from years of fighting the NHS. She tells me wearily that ITV has just been in to see her because the CQC has given the hospital the "all clear". She is not happy. In her opinion, there are still plenty of problems that need fixing.

Breaks Cafe is where Julie came after her mother died. She had never run a cafe before. But she and Bella had come here together. They had seen the lease up for rent. They had joked together about the idea of taking the lease and running the cafe together. So when her mother died it seemed like the right thing to do.

"Without the cafe it never would have worked," she says. In the years after 2007, Breaks Cafe became the centre of her campaign. In press photos taken at the time the campaign was at its height, you can see Julie, Ken Lowndes and others grouped for the photograph in the cafe with a huge banner saying "Cure the NHS" hung across the wall behind where I am sitting now.

We talk about her mother for a bit. She tells me what it was like moving back from living with her stepmother to be with her mother when she was a child.

"My mother was more working class than me. I had had a more middle-class upbringing, church on Sunday. With mum, there was no church, no TV. But everybody loved her. She was such a lovely character."

She tells me her mum threw herself into causes, was devoted to others and would take people in from the streets and feed them. "Really?" I ask, rather sceptically. "Literally!", she insists. "She would invite homeless people into the house at Christmas, who would sit there with you at dinner." She laughs and says it was "terrible". But her admiration shows and it seems to have acted as an inspiration to her.

Breaks Cafe became a place of refuge for people who could come in off the street and talk about what had happened to them or their relatives at the hospital. It became the unofficial place to which patients who were concerned about their care would come.

Every hospital trust in England is required to have a Patient Advice and Liaison Service. This is a group of people employed by the organisation to listen to the complaints and concerns of patients. You can probably imagine how well that works. At times, PALS can give the impression of having being created as the most efficient means of channelling patient complaints directly into the back of the bottom drawer of the filing cabinet in the furthest corner of the basement.

In Stafford, Julie made the local PALS service redundant by providing an alternative. Breaks Cafe was different. In Julie, patients knew they had someone on their side. By dint of her media profile, the hospital realised they could not ignore her. Patients could arrive, order a tea and explain their problems. Julie could then get on the phone to the medical director and start to deal with it.

This was unprecedented. This was a patient with real power. Beyond all the campaigning and the protesting and the arguing, this above all, is what Julie achieved. She created a moment when patients had real authority, when they could insist on being listened to, when the NHS knew there were real consequences if they did not pay attention to their opinions.

She reckons on more than one occasion she has saved a patient's life. She tells the story of a patient in Cannock Chase Hospital – a smaller community hospital run by the same management as Mid-Staffordshire. A woman came to the cafe saying her mother had gone into the hospital and had been put on nil-by-mouth for nine days while waiting for a swallowing test. "They have a well-known saying in Cannock – don't cough or they put you on nil-by-mouth," she says. The woman had come from the hospital after learning that her mother had now been put on an end-of-life care pathway without her knowledge and the drip was being turned off.

If she had made a complaint on the ward, she might well have been met with an "I'm in charge." But with Julie on her side it was different. Julie phoned the medical director. Within hours the patient was back on a drip and nursed back to strength before being discharged to a nursing home. "This was back in February," she says. Six months later and she is still doing fine.

The idea of "empowering patients" has been a consistent theme throughout all efforts to reform the NHS for several decades now. The idea is that patients have too little say about their own healthcare and that they should be more involved in the decisions about their care. For what might appear a relatively innocuous idea it is surprisingly contentious among many who work in healthcare.

In 2010, I was invited to speak in favour of this idea at a debate in London, the Battle of Ideas, along with a repre-sentative of the Patients Association and two GPs. Both GPs dismissed the idea as nothing more than a political gimmick, an idea foisted on the health service by politicians trying to curry favour with pushy middle-class people who wanted to try and squeeze more out of the system than was their due. The overwhelming majority of patients they saw, they said, had no desire to be asked to make choices. They wanted the doctor to make the decisions. After all, that was why the doctor had gone to medical school and not the patient.

The audience – young, metropolitan, intellectual – were clearly on the side of the GPs. My hopes of shifting the mood of the room were lifted briefly when a woman stood up and said that she was only alive today because she had researched her own illness and found out that a therapy was available in the UK that her GP did not know about. That should swing it, I thought. It did not. The majority still felt that giving patients more information and more control over how they were treated would simply create demands and burdens on the health service that were of little or no benefit to the majority. Patients did not want choice or control, it was something politicians talked about to garner popularity.

During the debate, the audience seemed to regard the GPs as a more authoritative voice for what patients wanted than the speaker from the Patients Association. Doctors have at times been effective defenders of patients' interests. But there are dangers if we see the medical professional as the representative of the patient. In surveys,* NHS patients express very high levels of satisfaction with their doctors, whether at the GP practice or at a hospital. But, compared to these overall levels of satisfaction, patients are less complimentary about how well doctors explain tests and treatments or involve patients in decisions about their care. When these ratings are compared to other countries, the NHS does not do well. In international surveys, the UK has been rated one of the worst countries for giving patients choices and involving them in decisions.† In most opinion polls, if patients are asked if they want to be able to make choices about their treatment, most say yes. That

---

* ENHS National Patient Survey programme.

† The Commonwealth Fund International Health Policy Surveys from 1998 to 2011 have placed the UK among the worst of the countries studied for involvement in shared decision making over most of that period. The two most recent surveys in 2010 and 2011, however, have shown a marked improvement as policies to encourage greater patient involvement in decision making have an effect.

is equally true of people who are affluent and people who are not.

But patients saying they want to have choices does not mean they are capable of making choices. The decisions are often rather complicated. One of the most telling comments made during the debate on patient choice was that expecting patients to make decisions about their care is unfair because: "It's not like buying cornflakes."

That sounds a little patronising. There are many situations in life where we rely on the guidance of experts. If my car breaks down, I take it to a mechanic who then explains to me what they plan to do and gets my permission. Maybe I do not know what a carburettor is. But I would still be miffed if the mechanic told me "It's a bit more complicated than buying cornflakes". The fact that a decision is complicated does not mean I lose either my right or my interest in being involved.

But the "it's more complicated than buying cornflakes" argument is often made as part of a rather convoluted and internal debate about the nature of patient choice.

There are two schools of thought that have advocated the idea of patients being more active in deciding what happens to them. The first is economic. The idea is that patients with more information and control over their healthcare can make healthcare providers compete for their business. This, it is hoped, will drive up standards. Much of the focus is on choosing *who* treats you.

The second argument for patient choice focusses much more on how to improve the experience of being cared for. This argument is put forward by patient rights advocates who want patients to have more control of *what* happens to them. They want doctors to be better at explaining the options and making sure that patients' views are not ignored.

The distinction is not that hard and fast – often decisions about *who* treats you and *what* treatment you get will overlap or indeed be the same. But the two lines of argument come from slightly different perspectives and bring different associations.

Much of the opposition to patient choice comes from those who are strongly opposed to the economic arguments. This is understandable. Patients capable of acting as independent consumers are few and far between. The notion of a "consumer" fails to capture the complexity of the relationship between a doctor and patient.

The Dutch academic Annemarie Mol has written at length on the subject. She argues that there is a fundamental conflict between what she calls the "logic of choice" and the "logic of caring". Caring involves taking responsibility for the person. Treating them as a "consumer" does not.

In her world of "caring", healthcare professionals treat the patient as a "crucial member of the care team". She describes how a carer does not leave a patient to make a choice, they carefully explain different possibilities to a patient, guide them through alternatives, help them make decisions but all the time being conscious of what their needs are, not just their wants. She tells us how they are "concerned with the specific problems of specific individuals in specific circumstances", and how they work out how the different people involved in the patient's care can "collaborate in order to improve, or stabilise, a person's situation".

Her description of the logic of caring is excellent. The odd thing about it is that is sets out almost exactly what many advocates of patient choice are calling for.

The ideal for a patient would be, as Mol describes, a healthcare professional who understands the different options available to a patient – the possible treatments, the ways in which that treatment might be delivered and the implications for the patient both clinical and non-clinical; who understands the patients needs and elicits their desires; who uses this information to recommend a suggested course of action; helps them to decide and who then co-ordinates activity to make sure it all happens.

I do not agree with her that the patient can be thought of as a "member of the care team". The patient is in quite a different position. The patient is the one who carries the consequences of every decision. That is why it is the patient who has the final say on what treatment they receive. The patient is – or rather should be – the captain of the team. But other than that, I think most people would whole-heartedly endorse the ideal she describes.

The bit I struggle with is the idea that consumerism should be opposed on the grounds that it fails to capture the richness of this ideal. Arguing against "choice" on the grounds that it falls short of "helping [patients] make decisions". It seems counter-productive when we are still so far from the ideal of informed patients engaged in the decisions about their care. Whatever the short-comings of consumerism, it has worked to some degree and has brought benefits.*

We need every lever we can use to try to encourage patients to take a more active role in the management of their care because the evidence is that in a significant number of patients, their preferences are never heard or are over-ridden. For example, we know that if the time is taken to properly explain to patients the advantages and risks of undergoing an operation, about one in five

---

* For an evaluation of choice in the English NHS see A Dixon et al., Patient Choice: how patients choose and how providers respond. King's Fund, 2010.

people choose not to have the operation. To be clear: one in five people who have operations have been persuaded to undergo surgery under a misapprehension.* As one colleague memorably put it, these people have not been operated on, they have been assaulted with a scalpel.

Take heart disease, for example. Patients with "stable angina" have a degree of chest pain caused by blocked arteries but are in no imminent danger of a heart attack. If drug therapies do not work, surgical interventions to unblock heart vessels can help alleviate the symptoms. But it is important to know that these interventions, which are not without risk, make no difference to your outcome. Your chances of having a heart attack or of dying or of needing to go to hospital are the same whether or not you have the operation. Unfortunately this is not always explained to the patient. When it is, the number agreeing to have the operation drops by twenty per cent.

The figures are even more dramatic for other procedures. For example, some studies have found forty per cent fewer patients opting for surgery on the prostate when they are in full possession of the facts.

---

* For a summary of the evidence on this and on the issue of doctors understanding of patient priorities see see A Mulley et al., Patients' Preferences Matter. King's Fund, 2012.

Indirect evidence that patient views are ignored comes from the very different rates of treatments at different hospitals and in different geographical areas. For example, your likelihood of having a hysterectomy for menstrual bleeding varies enormously from one part of the UK to another. When these figures are debated, there is often a strong chorus from doctors that the variations might just reflect doctors accurately understanding the preferences of their patients. Maybe. It could be true that the women of Kent, say, are unusually willing to be rid of their uterus compared to the women of Northumbria. But it seems unlikely.

Finally we have the evidence of surveys showing that what doctors think patients want is not what they want. Doctors asked to rate the top priorities for patients undergoing chemotherapy reckoned that extending life was the priority for 96 per cent of their patients. When the patients were asked only 59 per cent agreed. When doctors were asked what the priorities were for patients undergoing treatment for breast cancer, they said that retaining the breast was the priority for 71 per cent. When patients were asked the same question only 7 per cent said this was their priority.

This matters because it affects the way doctors make recommendations. In a brilliant if mischievous piece of research, Peter Ubel, a US doctor who has spent his life researching the ethics of medicine, sent questionnaires to representative samples of doctors. They were given scenarios in which a patient with prostate cancer had to opt for either a treatment with a low risk of death and a high risk of complications or one with a higher death rate but fewer complications. Some were asked what they would recommend. Others were asked what they would do if they were the patient. This produced two very different sets of results. The doctors were more likely to opt for the treatment with low complications but higher risk of death for themselves than they were to recommend it to their patients.*

So we are some way from the ideal that both choice advocates and, it would seem, their opponents hold out as the model of good healthcare. But is it really worth time and effort trying to fix the problem? Are there not more important things we should be doing with our scarce resources?

The anti-choice lobby says that giving patients a choice would add a burden to the healthcare service and the resources would be better used elsewhere. The

---

* PA Ubel et al., Physicians recommend different treatments for patients than they would choose for themselves. Archives of Internal Medicine, vol. 171, no. 7, 2011: 630–4. doi:10.1001/archinternmed.2011.91

pro-choice lobby points out that when you give patients more say over their own treatment they actually demand less intervention and take better care of themselves. So it not only makes patients happier, it more than pays for itself.

But I think there is one more very important reason why we need to give patients much greater control over what happens to them.

It is time now to go back to Andrew McAneney. When we left him, back in Newark, he was explaining how the one thing he wanted was somebody who was on his side. Somebody who would look out for him and make sure he got the treatment he needed. What Annemarie Mol would call a person following the "logic of care".

I said I thought his request very reasonable but that it was not something he would get. The reason I am doubtful is because I do not believe anyone is going to do this better than he, with the help of friends and family, has done himself. And I do not think he would settle for anything less than someone doing this with the same thoroughness that they bring to the task.

It is hard work. Trying to sort out getting Andrew the care he needs has taken perseverance and pestering, asking questions and checking. In the main, much of this energy has been spent fighting the system. If instead, they had simply got what they originally wanted – if Andrew had had his treatment when first referred – it would have been better for him and better for the health system.

Rather than holding out the promise of an NHS that will understand your needs and make sure you get what is necessary, it would be more realistic to recognise that, for a great many patients, the NHS will never understand their needs better than they do themselves. An NHS that gave them more authority – by making sure that they receive all the information about their care; by letting them, if they want, book tests and appointments; by enabling them to re-order prescriptions and medical supplies; and, yes, by encouraging them to take decisions about what treatments they receive, giving them opportunities to speak up and listening very carefully when they suspect things are going wrong – that would be an NHS far more likely to ensure that patients were well looked after.

When doctors say their patients do not want to make choices, it is important to recognise that the willingness of patients to make choices very much depends on how difficult or easy we make it for them. But they are right that the implication of giving patients choice and control, also means burdening them with decisions and responsibilities. We would all, of course, much prefer to be able to put our medical care in the hands of a system that can be relied upon to ensure that the right decisions are made and the right care is delivered.

The problem we have to deal with is that the right decisions will not get made and the right things will not happen without the patient being given greater say in the situation.

Angela Stubbs, like many other patients, is sceptical about being asked to take more control and responsibility for her healthcare.

Angela knows about being a patient. She has had plenty of practice over the last twenty years, during which she has had breast cancer, leukemia, non-Hodgkin's lymphoma as well as growths on her skin. She has seen more doctors in her life than anyone would ever want to but she always listens carefully to what they say and does what she is told.

Angela Stubbs is my mother-in-law. We are sitting together discussing her health after a lunch to celebrate her 50th wedding anniversary. Her eldest daughter has come across from Australia. My wife and I are there along with my brother-in-law and his wife. The grandchildren are behaving themselves.

She has enjoyed the occasion and is coping well with eating in spite of the lymphoedema that has swollen her left hand and arm, making it impossible to move them. It is only one of the many symptoms of her breast cancer but it is particularly trying. Two years ago she was playing tennis. Now she finds it hard to get out of a chair. Her passion for gardening has also been rather curtailed by this latest development.

I think she may be worried that I want her to complain about the way she has been treated. She does not want to. She feels that in the main things have been managed extremely well.

When she talks about her doctors she is hesitant to ever criticise and when she does say something less than positive usually follows it with: "but they are so busy, so busy" to make clear that she understands how hard it is for them and how unreasonable it is for her to expect more.

She is also very busy herself. The day-to-day tasks of getting up and getting dressed take longer now and require the help of Michael, her husband. He has to see to the wound dressings each day. There are the medications to take and keep track of. And most days there is at least one appointment, either at the hospital or one of the clinics she attends.

The breast cancer was first discovered eighteen years ago and was successfully treated. But now it has come back suddenly and rather aggressively. She had an operation in 2010 and they took out as much as they could.

Friends suggested she should consider treatment outside Cornwall, where she lives, but she did not like the idea. She likes the people who look after her in Truro. She could not, by any stretch of the imagination, be described as a pushy patient. When I ask her what she would like to have been different she has to think for quite a long time before answering. But her main observation is that: "You have to be alert."

She gives the example of the tests she is supposed to have periodically while she is on Herceptin. If she does not keep tabs herself and remind people, they can get missed.

And she is troubled by the thought that other things might have been missed – in particular, whether the lymphoedema could have been prevented.

Like most patients, Angela feels no great need for the way medicine is practiced to be changed. The task of managing her illness is an enormous burden and the idea that she might want to take on more control of her care or more responsibility for what happens to her is hardly an appealing offer.

But she and Michael know her situation better than anyone else. They are the only people who talk to the haematologist, the oncologist, the lymphoedema nurse, the staff at the clinic where she goes for chemotherapy, the nurse who visits her and her GP. They are the only people who have the complete picture of what is happening.

So when she has a sense of unease about the way her treatment is being managed, or if she wants to change the way things are done, her views should carry real weight and consequence.

It is in this sense that the patient should never be seen as "part of the team". They are in charge of the whole operation. Doctors may complain that patients are not very good at being the boss – they are often ill-informed, they may at times have some pretty wrong-headed views about what needs to happen – but it is their life and their every word should be given its due. The role of the doctors and nurses is to help them do this.

Patients may be ill-informed about medicine but they make up for this by being extremely well informed about themselves. As a result, they are right much more often than you might have thought. Take, for example, patients who ask for a second opinion. Often patients are reluctant to do this because if feels like trouble-making. In fact they are helping themselves and the whole health system.

Getting the wrong diagnosis is dangerous for the patient and wastes the doctor's time. Patients have a good sense of when they suspect a diagnosis is not right. When this was looked at in the US among breast cancer patients they found that the majority of those who asked for a second opinion were right to have their doubts – the original diagnosis had been wrong.*

Encouraging patients to speak up and giving them a greater say over how their care is managed will not make life harder for doctors. It will make life easier. It is the patient whose life will be made less easy. But for the opportunity to make sure their care is right, it is probably a fair trade.

In the end, the sense in which the patient is in charge only really becomes clear when medical opinion is not there to guide you. We will be lucky if all decisions about our medical care are so straightforward that we can simply rely on the advice of doctors. Often we will be unaware of the extent to which we are doing this. But occasionally, the reality of where responsibility lies is laid bare.

Jill Maben knows how tough it can be looking after patients. She began her working life as a staff nurse in a hospital in Dulwich before quickly getting burned out and deciding to quit. After a period of study and travel she ended up working once more as a nurse in Australia and

---

* This study in Michigan by Michael Sabel used a multi-disciplinary team to review patient notes. It should be pointed out that review by a multi-disciplinary team is standard practice in the NHS for cancer patients but not for other areas of medicine. The point remains that the patients who sought a second opinion were found to have good reason. Studies of misdiagnosis show rates of between 6–12 per cent generally, whereas rates among patients that initiated second opinions range from 30 per cent to over 50 per cent.

found her vocation again. She is now Professor of Nursing at King's College in London where she works on designing the right working environment to allow clinical staff to provide high quality compassionate care.

Jill's son George was only two years old when he was diagnosed with a hypothalamic hamartoma. The doctors at Great Ormond Street spelt out for Jill and her partner Robert Mead what this meant. A hypothalamic hamartoma is a rare condition in which a small lump (benign tumour) in the brain causes unintended neural discharges. In time, this epileptic activity leads to seizures, known as gelastic or laughing seizures. The seizures, they were told, would become more and more severe, George's mental development would be affected and his quality of life would gradually deteriorate. "The best you can hope for is that someone in George's life time comes up with a cure" they were told.

Being a nurse and a researcher, Jill went straight to the British Library and read every piece of research published about hypothalamic hamartomas. It was one of the worst days of her life. Wherever she looked the conclusion was the same. People had attempted to operate but the results had been disastrous. There was no cure. The only option was to work through the various drug treatments and try to find the combination that was most effective at limiting the progression of the illness.

As time passed, life did not get any easier. George struggled to learn, he became withdrawn and would not socialise, hiding inside his jumper when visitors came. His behaviour became obsessive and at times challenging, insisting on switching lights on and off or watching the washing machine spin round for hour after hour.

It was the internet that first opened up new possibilities. One day Jill put up a post on an epilepsy website describing her son's diagnosis and asking if anyone else out there was going through the same situation. For months there was no response and she had almost forgotten about it when an email popped up from someone in the US inviting her to join a web forum for families with children with George's condition. She was the seventh person to sign up.

It was through this group that she first learned of Jeffrey Rosenfeld, a surgeon in Melbourne, who was developing new approach to operating on hypothalamic hamartomas. Conventional wisdom argued that, when operating on the brain, the surgeon should always take the shortest route to the tumour. In the case of hypothalamic hamartomas, that meant going in behind the eyes. But the problem was it made it hard for the surgeons to see what they were doing. The high levels of damage this causes to the patient meant that most doctors abandoned the procedure as a viable form of treatment.

Rosenfeld had developed an alternative approach, going in through the top of the head. He was getting good results. Jill decided to find out more. She had copies of George's MRI scans so she sent them to Australia. When the doctors wrote back to say they believed they could achieve a 95 per cent removal without side effects and leave George free of seizures, she burst into tears. Partly it was the relief of hearing someone for the first time hold out hope. But in that same moment, she understood the awful responsibility that this message had presented her with.

She spoke to the neurologist in Melbourne – making a recording of the conversation so that she could play it back to friends and family and get their views. The call was encouraging so she decided to seek the advice of her doctors at Great Ormond Street. This did not go well.

She was referred to a surgeon who told her that the Australian approach was experimental and that it was "too risky". Jill and Rob were knocked back by this. Jill understood how new the technique was. She had read all the research. She knew the risks and yet it still struck her as possibly the best option for George. She could not understand how the surgeon was coming to such a different conclusion and felt able to talk so categorically about it. They felt they were being told they were irresponsible. It got worse when he then recommended instead that they try a French radiotherapy treatment. Why was French radiotherapy not under discussion before? Why, now that she was considering something that the consultants had not mentioned, were they coming up with new ideas?

At this point, she says, they felt very, very alone. Should they take the advice of George's doctors in England and ignore what was being held out as perhaps their son's best hope? Or should they act on the assurances of the Australian doctors and fly George half way round the world for an operation that everyone agreed was experimental?

In the end it was the patients that made the difference. She called the Australian team back and said she would like to talk to other patients who had been through what she was going through. The doctors in Australia contacted other patients and put her in touch with them. In particular, one mother who had also trained as a nurse was able to talk to her about the attitude and approach of the Melbourne team. Like Jill, she said, she had been worried. She thought that they might be using her child to further their research careers. But as she got to know them, she had come to the view that they only had her and her child's interests at heart.

For Jill, understanding their motivation was just as important as understanding the technical skills. Trust is important. She had to weigh up on the one hand the risks posed by George's rapidly deteriorating condition and, on the other, the risks of undergoing surgery that could prove fatal. She was very aware of the need to be able to live with the decision whatever the outcome. It was the testimony of the patients, rather than the competing expert opinions of leading doctors, that gave her the confidence to make the decision to go to Australia.

There is a photograph of Jill with Rob and their baby daughter having a picnic on a piece of grass outside the hospital in Melbourne. They picked the spot because you can see the building where the operating theatre is situated. George is inside undergoing six hours of surgery. Jill's face is unrecognisable, drawn with stress and anxiety.

Jill shows me a different photo. It is picture of George as he is today. A twenty-year-old man, smartly dressed in a suit, dark curls to his shoulders and a huge smile. Following the operation it took some time for George to recover. But the seizures stopped and never came back. He never recaptured the lost years of development. But his life today is unrecognisable from the prognosis held out for him when he was two. He is sociable and active. He has friends and interests. He has hope and opportunities in place of an inevitable path of deterioration.

One of the fears that doctors have of patient choice is that it will undermine trust. Trust is rooted in their authority, it is argued. If the patient is in charge, the doctor has no authority and trust is undermined.

Some doctors are unclear how they are supposed to talk to patients if the patient is the one making the decision. If patients ask them to make a decision, should they agree? And if the patient does not like their advice, what should they do?

The best suggestion I can make is to try to imagine that the patient is your new chief executive. He or she understands very little right now, but there is every likelihood that in time they will understand everything. How would you behave in that situation? If they ask you to make a decision on their behalf, you would probably want to ask a few questions and try to ensure that whatever you advised, would suit them. If they looked puzzled or uncertain of your advice, you might want to try to elicit more. If they expressed a view, you would take it very seriously into consideration. And you would probably want to hold back from suggesting that their preferred course of action was in some ways irresponsible except in those moments when you were on very firm ground. In other words you would want to treat them with respect – as someone who may not possess all the knowledge – but who certainly has authority.

A doctor's authority rests on technical expertise. The patient's authority rests on the fact that they have the final say. In Jill's case, it was what other patients said that was the deciding factor. The doctors were the experts in medicine. But the patients were the experts in which doctors you should place your trust in. And every patient has to make that decision.

CHAPTER 11

Where is the love?

The comedian Marlon Davis has a sketch in which he laments the inadequate relationship he has with "his doctor".

> "All my life I've been filling in forms asking me who my doctor is. Every time I write down the same information. But I ain't seen the guy since I was about three years old. Every time I go to see my doctor, I get shown into this room and someone I have never seen before says, 'Can I help you?' I say, 'Yeah, you can help me. You can tell me what happened to my doctor?'"

It is a common complaint. Many patients feel that there is no-one in the health service who is "their" doctor – someone who is on their side and who knows them personally. It is something every patient wants but few get. At its worst, this lack of personal connection with the people looking after us can turn into something much more chilling – the sense that no-one cares.

Each year, the Patients Association publishes a selection of stories about patients whose care has catastrophically failed. They are similar to the stories told to the Mid-Stafford-shire Independent Inquiry, and to some of the complaints reported by the Health Services Ombudsman. The elements are familiar: patients left in pain; patients not helped to go to the toilet; patients not helped to eat; patients not told what is going on or having their views ignored.

Some of these stories culminate in degrading experiences for patients left in filthy beds and ignored. Others end more seriously, with the patient's death caused by basic errors made in the face of protests from the patient or their families.

Because the NHS is a national organisation, each of these stories does not simply reflect on the particular organisation caring for the patient. They are national stories and they are seen to reflect on the whole of our health system. In France, a scandal in a hospital in Lyons might be a story of interest only to the people of the area. In England, a scandal in the NHS is something that everybody cares about. These stories prompt real disquiet.

But they do little to prompt support for NHS reform. This is because many elements of government policy on the

NHS seems irrelevant to this issue. Indeed some aspects of it can at times seem to be exacerbating it.

If what we all want is doctors and nurses who care about us, it is hard to see how much of the effort to reform the NHS will help to achieve this. Centralising hospital services seems to make them more distant rather than more caring. Asking doctors to get involved in managing budgets seems to take them further away from being the champions of the patient. Asking patients to be more involved in their care can feel like more of the burden is shifted onto their shoulders.

The drive to make healthcare more efficient and more reliable has had a cost for patients. Hospital procedures can become more streamlined and medical teams more specialised but the only thing that does not get more efficient, more specialised and more streamlined in all of this is you and I – the patient. Indeed, quite the opposite is happening. As patients, we are becoming more complex and more differentiated in our needs. Today most NHS patients are older people, with more than one illness and little or no prospect of their conditions being "cured". They are signing on to receive healthcare for the rest of their lives.

Making healthcare more efficient and more reliable brings benefits. But it has also resulted in many patients feeling a lack of any joined-up approach to their care. The continuity of having one person who knows you – whether that's the midwife, the social care worker or the GP – has been sacrificed for the efficiency of having greater flexibility in the way staff are scheduled.

When scandals such as the events at Mid-Staffordshire come to light, the gulf between our ideals and the way in which care staff are found to have behaved is shocking. It is sobering to discover how professional carers can, at times, demonstrate what appear to be astonishing levels of callousness towards patients.

Kane Gorny, a twenty two year old from South London, died of dehydration on a ward in St George's Hospital, a major teaching hospital, after both he and his mother pleaded with nurses for hours to give him a drink. Gorny was suffering from diabetes insipidus which meant he needed medication to enable his body to retain fluid. His mother, aware of the risks, had repeatedly informed staff of the importance of the medication and assumed it was being dealt with. Gorny, in a confused state after his operation, did not understand that he was not being given the correct medicine. The nurses did not know he needed it. The mother's words were ignored – after all, instructions to administer medicines come from the doctor, not from the patient's mother. But the surgeon had not read the patients notes and so had given no instruction. In desperation, as his condition weakened, Gorny called 999 and the police arrived but hospital staff sent them away again. Shortly after that, he died.

In delivering her verdict, the coroner concluded that Kane was "let down by incompetence of staff, poor communication, lack of leadership, both medical and nursing, a culture of assumption." Each individual step in the chain of events that led to his death would, in other circumstances, might have been of only modest concern. It sometimes happens that information about a patient's medication requirements are not communicated to the nurses on the ward. It sometimes happens that the complaints of patients and their carers get ignored. It is when these things coincide to cause someone's death that the full implications of such behaviour are exposed.

There is no point in blaming Gorny's death on the individual doctors and nurses involved. Such failures are an inevitable consequence of the way we run health services and it is this that needs to change. However there is something particularly horrifying about the idea of being under the care of nurses who have ceased to respond to your cries for help. It is, quite literally, the stuff of nightmares.

Such stories prompted both the current Prime Minister and the last to commission reports into how to improve nursing standards. Gordon Brown established a Commission on the Future of Nursing and Midwifery in England which reported in 2010. In 2011 David Cameron established the Nursing and Care Quality Forum to provide further ideas.

There is some common ground between the 2009 report and the initial recommendations of the *Forum*. Both call for greater accountability for nurse leaders – from ward sisters and matrons upwards – and greater efforts to measure the quality of nursing care.

The *Forum* stressed the need to think about nurse staffing levels and to use feedback from patients to understand what it was like for them. They also recommended paying more attention to one of the most telling pieces of information about NHS services. Each year the NHS conducts a survey of staff and includes a question on whether or not they would be happy to have a relative or spouse treated at the organisation where they work. At some hospitals, the majority would not. The *Forum* rightly suggested that all NHS organisations should aim to provide a level of service which its own staff is willing to use.

There is also long-overdue recognition that not everyone is cut out to be a carer. The *Forum* recommended that nurses should be recruited on the basis that they have the right emotional make up – a "caring nature" – as much as for their technical skills. Tolerating people who do the job badly is not acceptable if it means patients are harmed. Something of a turning point came in 2010 when the president of the Royal College of Nurses, Andrea Spyropoulos, called on her members to expose bad nurses.

Better training can also help, and much can be learned from organisations outside healthcare. There are coffee chains that have more rigorous systems to ensure their staff behaves in a polite and conciliatory manner to customers than parts of the NHS.

The least convincing responses to the so-called "crisis in compassion" have been the various grandiose statements of intent. The NHS Constitution in England and the Charter of Patient Rights and Responsibilities in Scotland are both attempts to set down the standards that the public should expect in the hope that this might make it so.

They are remarkably empty documents and only emphasise how weak the rights of patients are. For example, you have the "right to expect" your local NHS to provide the services it considers "necessary" – or in plain English, the right to get what you are given.

Both documents also include the right to be treated appropriately, although the words do little to give confidence. The NHS constitution says you "have the right to be treated with dignity and respect, in accordance with your human rights". It is hard to know what that means beyond a promise not to torture or wrongly imprison you. It certainly seems to fall short of providing legal grounds to end the indignities some patients have suffered.

Although these documents seem light on substance, strengthening patients' rights can offer a way to afford people greater protection. The one consistent element throughout all the stories of failure and tragedy is the position of powerlessness patients have been put in. Lack of respect shown to patients is a painful reflection of how little authority they have. Julie Bailey's account of the seven weeks she spent in Mid-Staffordshire Hospital is a catalogue of the many ways a patient can be snubbed, ignored, spoken to rudely, blamed for things that are not their fault, disbelieved and lied to.*

Stronger rights to have complaints independently reviewed would be helpful. As would a right to some form of compensation proportionate to the level of humiliation suffered when, for example, a patient is left untended through the night.

Consent is another process that can be used to strengthen the authority of patients. For much of healthcare, the process of consenting patients has become perfunctory to the point of being a formality. In some cases

---

* J Bailey, From the Ward to Whitehall. 2012.

that is understandable. If the patient is having a routine treatment for a common problem, the legal process of consent may seem overly bureaucratic.

Perhaps because of this attitude, we now find ourselves in the astonishing situation of people claiming that patients have been put on an end-of-life care pathway without either being told that this was happening or agreeing to it. The claims are plausible, not least as the national audits of end-of-life care revealed gaps in documentation around the information given to patients.*

An end-of-life care pathway is a series of steps designed to ensure that patients have a comfortable, dignified and pain-free death. It is a well thought through process that covers all the important aspects such as pain control, stopping resuscitation and withdrawing artificial support.

The pathway states that patients, where possible, and family members or carers should always be consulted about the decision to put a patient on the pathway. But the decision itself is taken by the medical staff. Strictly speaking, there is no legal obligation to have patient consent since this decision is not itself an intervention but is rather a framework for deciding a series of actions, such as withdrawal of artificial life support and management of pain.

---

* National Care of the Dying Audit – Hospitals (NCDAH), Round 3: www.rcplondon.ac.uk www.rcplondon.ac.uk

Managed correctly, end-of-life care should involve continuous monitoring of the patient's condition, determining at each stage the appropriate level of pain control, nutrition and hydration to leave them comfortable and to allow the process of dying to be as dignified as possible. Done wrong, it can appear tantamount to simply ordering the patient's death by withdrawing support. The difference is partly in the skill and compassion with which the process is managed. But it is mainly in the extent to which the patient and their relatives are informed about what is happening and are involved in all decisions. This is essential because decisions about end-of-life care are based on the doctor's assessment of whether or not the patient is in the process of dying. Such assessments are inevitably fallible – as demonstrated by the fact that patients have been assessed as dying put on an end-of-life care pathway and then rallied. In this situation, it is essential to monitor the situation closely and keep all concerned informed throughout. Of course there may be circumstances where the patient explicitly does not wish to know. But for the many patients and families who do want to know, it is hard to think of anything that shows a greater lack of respect than the failure to do this.

Being treated with respect does not mean simply that people are not rude to you. It also means that people do not withhold information from you or make life and death decisions about you without talking to you first.

By all accounts, Harold Shipman was rather popular with his patients and had an excellent bedside manner. His charm rather wore off when it was discovered that he was also the UK's most prolific serial killer, estimated to have killed over 250 of his patients.

Dr Amir Hannan was the man who shouldered the unenviable task of taking on Harold Shipman's practice in Hyde, Manchester, after Shipman's conviction and death. He needed from the outset to do something that would restore trust. He needed to find some way of demonstrating that nothing like that could ever happen again. The way he decided to do this was to try to turn on its head the relationship between patient and doctor. And the cornerstone of this was to give his patients access to all the information he had about them and to start helping them make use of it. All of them. Including Margaret Rickson, who at 80 years of age gave talks with Amir explaining the benefits of being able to use her own medical record.

Providing stronger rights to information is a promising way to give patients greater authority. In theory, patients already have the right to access their medical records. But it is a largely empty right, as it does not enable you to get the information you want at the moment you need it and in a format you can understand. What patients need is access to the same electronic information that doctors have.

Information technology has the potential to transform medicine. Electronic health records can be used to accurately communicate information between members of a care team, to make sure that tasks are performed at the right time, to ensure that warning signs are not missed and to audit the quality of care.* In well-run hospitals, most information about patients will be recorded on electronic systems. These records can then be scanned for problems that the nurse or doctor might not have picked up. Some systems are capable of sending out an alert if the patient's condition is deteriorating. Algorithms can be run over the data to check whether the patient's course of treatment complies with recommendations. Decision aids can automatically prompt the doctor to consider alternative diagnoses or prescriptions on the basis of the information recorded.

However, despite the vast potential for information technology to improve healthcare, its implementation to date has been disappointing. Part of the reason for this is that too little has been done to involve the patient. As a result, electronic patient records and computerisation are

---

* See for example T Lee and J Mongan, Chaos and Organisation in Health Care. MIT Press, 2009.

sometimes seen as barriers to good care, rather than aids. Technology can be seen as a further mechanism by which the personal aspects of care are reduced.

American doctor and author Abraham Verghese[*] has seen it happening in US hospitals, where electronic patient records are more widely used than in the UK. He has a wonderful description of the "i-patient" – the scans and test data that represent the patient on the screen – becoming more real than the actual physical patient. "The i-patient is getting wonderful care all across America," he says. Meanwhile, "The real patient often wonders 'Where is everyone? When are they going to come by and explain things to me? Who is in charge?'"

One way to address this is to make sure that the patient has just as much access to the i-patient as the doctor. They too should be able to see all the information and scans on the system. Better still they should be able to see it in formats that are easily intelligible and which they can use in a range of settings and applications. If the data is used to tell the doctor whether the treatment conforms with recommendations, it should do exactly the same for the patient. If the doctor sees prompts for alternative diagnoses, so should the patient.

---

[*]   Are computers getting between you and your doctor, The Atlantic, 6 June 2012.

Many of the stories of patients being disrespected and ignored occur when patients try to remind healthcare professionals about what they think needs to happen. For example, on the ward round the doctor might have said the patient should have a medication four times a day. If eight hours later this has not happened, the patient may become anxious. They may try to communicate with medical staff.

These situations can become strained for many reasons. The patient may feel unsure of themselves – after all the doctor might have changed the prescription later on away from the bedside. The professionals caring for them may take their comments as a criticism and respond negatively. Many things can contribute to the problem: lack of time in understaffed units; the mistaken belief that somebody else is doing something; or difficulties communicating because patient and professional do not share a common first language.

Your life as a patient may depend upon not being misunderstood. It may depend upon your words not being treated as additional information that needs to be taken into account by professionals making judgments about how to treat you but rather as the single most important voice of authority in determining what happens to you.

Real time electronic medical records shared between patient and carer have an important role to play in ending any such confusion. They have the potential to make it much harder to ignore what patients are saying by enabling them to see what is decided about them and to respond. If patients are informed about what should be happening, they can help ensure it does happen.

If medical records are so useful to patients, it might reasonably be asked why so few bother to get hold of them through the routes that are now available to them. But the routes available to patients now are, in the main, cumbersome and only worth pursuing if there is a major point of contention.

Patient access to medical records means making them as accessible as an online bank account or an online diary. It means making them available in ways that are immediately useful – useful to patients for whom the idea of being an empowered patient is not something that immediately appeals. Patients such as my mother-in-law.

As I sat talking to Angela Stubbs about her medical treatment, she wanted to explain the order of various events, so took out a well-used Letts diary with pencil notes on each page detailing information about clinics and her treatment. She had kept a record in order to help her keep track of the many things that were happening. As she leafed through it trying to check whether she had remembered the details correctly, I asked her whether it would be helpful if she could just look up her history on her computer. She nodded and agreed that this might indeed be rather useful. The fact that she has to keep pencil notes in a diary and struggle to recall which treatments have been prescribed to her at different times is an absurdity.

There is a huge amount of work that needs doing to transform medical records designed for doctors into information and applications designed to help patients manage their care. The technology is still in its infancy, but the first step to achieving this is ensuring that patients can access up-to-date electronic data about themselves.

In England the NHS has committed to do this. If delivered in the right way, it will enable the creation of new services, such as PatientsLikeMe, a web site that enables people to share information about themselves and learn from each other. Such services hold out the potential for patient groups to grow much stronger in their ability to support each other and find a collective voice for what they want.

Second opinion services may also start develop. Private insurance policies now offer second opinion services whereby you can elect to have your records and test results sent to another doctor who will review them and either confirm or suggest alternative diagnoses or treatment options. These second opinions are sought not just from doctors in the UK but internationally.* If NHS patients were to have access to their full NHS records, there is no reason why such options should not also be open to them.

Electronic patient records currently consist of all the information that doctors feel is necessary to manage the patient. But in time, it is to be hoped that they might also include the information that the patient wishes to be included. Information, for example, about their state of mind as much as their state of health. Or they may feel that information about the practical day-to-day challenges they face should be as much part of their record as their blood test data and prescription history.

A common objection to more widespread use of personal access to technology in healthcare is the fear that it will disadvantage those with less access. It is right to protect those at risk of this but not by slowing or discouraging technological development.

The biggest obstacle to personal technology in health is inertia. Healthcare systems have had great difficulty putting in place data recording systems which work and which doctors, nurses and audit clerks will use. In the US, healthcare providers are now financially incentivised to make "meaningful use" of electronic patient records,

---

* For example, Second Opinion Telemedicine Network and Chartis Insurance.

because without this added incentive it was simply too much bother.

The development of personal technology in health has been slow in large degree because the information needed to fuel the development of applications has been held within healthcare organisations that have shown little interest in the creation of new applications that would be of benefit to patients. By improving access to data there is every prospect that such technologies will prove one of the most powerful ways of ensuring that patients are safely looked after and their voices are heard.

Technology can be a way of helping patients influence the way healthcare is delivered rather than a barrier to personalised and improved care. It can help to create the relationship with healthcare professionals that so many patients crave – doctors that *do* know them and understand their wishes.

The information that might have kept Kane Gorny alive was on his medical records and in his head. No-one paid any attention to his or his mother's words. The desperation in his face somehow failed to communicate the urgency of the situation. The i-patient, however, might have been believed. Had he been able to call upon the testimony of the i-patient in his support, he might yet have lived.

CHAPTER 12

Everybody loses, everybody wins

Re-reading through the previous chapters, I am a bit worried that this book may come across as something of a downer. It might sound as though nobody is going to get what they want.

Patients would like somebody they can trust to understand their health needs and to make sure they get addressed. I think they are going to be disappointed. They are going to find they have plenty of doctors who understand particular aspects of their health, but no-one who understands everything. There will be plenty of people trying to make sure their needs get addressed, but they will be working in a system that has proved itself unreliable. As our health needs increase and become more complex, the disappointment will grow. The best many will be offered is the opportunity to take on more of the work of co-ordinating their care themselves.

Doctors would like to be left in peace to get on with looking after their patients. They do not want to be dragged into the difficult business of deciding how health services are run and how the money gets spent. But they will find themselves pulled more and more into the world that most of us inhabit, with annual appraisals, performance metrics and management objectives. They are going to find their every decision scrutinised by both doctors and accountants – or perhaps even by a doctor who understands finance. Some will fight it tooth and nail. Other will decide it is better to do the managing than be managed.

Communities are, on the whole, happy with their local health services the way they are. They are sceptical of the need to close A&E departments and move care into specialised centres. They are ambivalent at best about the idea of new services from private organisations (even if the people who use them are delighted with them). But whatever public opinion has to say on the matter, in an NHS where the finances are squeezed, the pace of such change is likely to accelerate. More and more services will either be centralised or moved into the community. A range of new businesses – some charitable, some for profit – will start to provide services.

These are all areas where the policies being enacted have been widely endorsed by those who work in the area of NHS policy. But they have failed to gain full acceptance even among NHS staff, let alone among the wider public.

It is true that in some opinion polls people are positive about some of these ideas, depending on how the question is phrased. Many people agree in principle that the NHS needs to change. Some notions, such as "choice", are popular in an abstract sense, even if less so in reality. But little in the reform agenda really resonates with the public.

You do not hear people in the pub complaining that no-one has shut down the dreadful local cancer clinic because of its poor outcomes; or bemoaning the shocking lack of engagement by the medical profession in fixing the financial problems facing the NHS. You might occasionally find someone in the corner complaining that the whole NHS should be handed over to the private sector. But you will probably want to steer well clear of them as they slump against the bar after six large gins. In any event, their voices will be drowned out by the cries from the other end of the bar that all the NHS needs is more money.

The policies that address the economics of healthcare are not policies that have captured the hearts and minds of the public. This is the tension that underlies the political debate. Those opposed to reform face economic forces which, like tectonic plates, tend, in the long run, to crush anything that stands in their way. Those in favour of reform face an indifferent or often hostile response from large sections of the profession and the public.

The result is a sort of policy "groundhog day" in which governments enact reforms which fail to get traction out in the real world and fail to produce the hoped for improvements. They respond to this with a new set of reforms that appear to the untrained eye to be little more than a rehashing of the last set of reforms.

The political shenanigans over the Health and Social Care Act have, in the main, been unhelpful. A largely unnecessary piece of legislation encompassing a largely unnecessary re-organisation of NHS structures, the act has been more of a distraction than a help in finding ways to make the NHS more sustainable. But the debate has been a salutary reminder, if any was needed, of just how much work is needed if the reform lobby are to persuade the country of the benefits of doing things differently.

Frustration at the difficulty of reforming the NHS is apparent wherever leaders of the healthcare industry gather. On the way in to one such event recently, I bumped into one of the country's most eminent doctors, who said wearily that it is so frustrating that we know exactly what *needs* to happen with our health services but somehow cannot *make* it happen. The event, held over breakfast in a downstairs room in the House of Commons, was attended by politicians from left and right, academics, industry leaders and medical experts. There were differences of opinion, to be sure. But the things that united them – the deeply held conviction that the NHS has to change and despondency at the pace with which it is possible the make this happen – were stronger.

As a group, they shared a belief that the ability of a society to look after the health of its citizens and to care for each other through infirm old age is the mark of a civilised society; that we have failed to always live up to that principle; that this is a problem of success rather than failure; that the cost of healthcare is not a burden but one of the most productive and beneficial things that we can do with the resources available to us and that this will only increase as medicine continues to make new discoveries.

We fear that the system is not working as it should. Too often it lets patients down. It is failing to identify the best ways to manage patients. It is failing to achieve the right balance of responsibility and authority between doctors and patients.

Somehow we have reached a point where the NHS has the power to destroy a brain tumour with radiation and replace a malfunctioning heart with an artificial one. Yet at the same time it is capable of leaving a patient crying in agony all night because there is no-one available to provide pain control; or letting them die because of an error on a prescription. The progress of medical science has been impressive. Progress in medical practice has proved much more elusive.

Efforts at reform to address this problem often face ambivalence among the medical profession. Some support the need for change. Others are creating new political parties to challenge them. The opponents of change tend to have less influence in government but a powerful voice in the public debate. This presents a challenge to politicians, as doctors are among the most trusted people in the country and politicians among the least.

The trust accorded to doctors and withheld from politicians is more a reflection of their roles than their moral character. Trust in politicians will always be low because politics is the stuff we do not agree about. Their job is to argue and compromise; to say things we disagree with or to fail to deliver the things we do agree with. It is no great surprise we think them untrustworthy. Doctors, in contrast, are there to look after us when we are in need. That is why we trust them. Whether the latest scandal is MPs fiddling their expenses or surgeons killing patients, doctors will always be more trusted. This gives them great influence.

Whenever professionals express views about how their work should be regulated or paid for, they bring to the debate the expertise that comes with doing the job along with a bias that comes from having a stake in the way things are organised. Doctors are, on the whole, given the benefit of the doubt, so that when they say things about how the NHS should work, their words carry great weight. However, the medical profession, like all professions, tends to be more effective at saying what it is opposed to than in leading calls for change. The net effect is a slowing down of the pace at which reforms can be implemented.

Poor execution has undermined aspects of the various reform programmes that have been implemented over the last decade The potential benefits of electronic patient records are well documented. But the initiatives to implement electronic patient records have rarely come close to delivering that potential. The promise of innovation from the private sector is yet to be properly fulfilled. Failure to always test whether re-configuration of services has actually made them better has undermined claims that these changes are being done for the good of patients.

Attempts to integrate care around the patient – for example providing more care at home or in local clinics, making use of telemedicine, or educating the patient in their own care – have had mixed results. Some efforts have worked well; in particular, initiatives that encourage patients to take a more active role in looking after themselves.* But in general, integration has yielded fewer benefits than hoped for.†

Greater accountability – through quality measurement and transparency – has been successful in driving up standards of care.‡ But the provision of this sort of information to patients has had only a limited impact on how they behave. The way the information is presented is often too technical and detailed for patients to make head or tail of it. Too often, there is no-one who will speak plainly about what complex statistics imply in terms of the options available for patients and the standards of care provided.

But, perhaps the biggest obstacle to reform of the NHS is the fact that the benefits to patients often seem rather abstract and intangible. The downside to change is often more obvious than the upside. In what way is care going to be better if my local services are rearranged? Why will anything be improved if I am given access to my medical

---

* A Kennedy et al., The effectiveness and cost effectiveness of a national lay-led self-care support programme for patients with long-term conditions: a pragmatic randomised controlled trial. Journal of Epidemiology & Community Health, vol. 61, no. 3, 2007: 254–61.

† National evaluation of Department of Health's integrated care pilots. Ernst & Young, RAND Europe and the University of Cambridge, March 2012.

‡ PG Shekelle et al., Does Public Release of Performance Results Improve Quality of Care? A systematic review. Health Foundation, 2008.

records? How would any of these reforms make my life any better?

Let me try and describe an ideal scenario. Let me begin with what will, in time, happen as a result of having access to your medical record.

From your phone, tablet or computer you will be able to read everything that has been noted or done about your health in a form that is understandable. It will describe the history of your symptoms, diagnoses, prescriptions and treatments. You will be able to add to it – indeed you will be expected to – updating information about your symptoms and your state of health.

You will be able to share it with others to alert them to concerns. You will use it to seek advice from both professionals and patients. It will enable you to automatically find other people in similar situations to ask their opinion. If you want to, you will be able to feed it into applications that generate lifestyle recommendations or identify possible issues with your regimen such as drug interactions. Other applications may compare your treatment to the treatment of other patients in similar situations, propose potential diagnoses or suggest alternative treatments. All of which you could discuss with your doctors.

It will detail any agreed programme of care and any steps you have agreed to take to look after yourself. You will use it to check whether these things are happening; to see what needs to be arranged; to book appointments; to make sure that test results have been received and viewed before you go to see the doctor; and to order repeat prescriptions or additional supplies such as wound dressings or colostomy bags.

The nature of treatment will change. You and those who care for you will find you are invited to attend education sessions as much as treatment sessions. The role of doctor will become increasingly that of expert adviser to help you in the management of your own health. Nurses and care workers will become as important if not more important than doctors for many patients. You will very likely find that you have a number of doctors who are expert in their areas of knowledge but none of whom understand in detail all the issues that affect your health.

You may not have anyone you would describe as "your doctor'". However you will have access to a medical service that knows who you are and can put you in contact with whoever you need – by phone, online or in person – twenty-four hours a day, seven days a week.

That might sound like a lot of work for the patient. How can we ask this of people who are unwell? Of course, many patients will not be in a position to do any of these things. But growing numbers will. For those that can, there will be a trade-off: more work on their part, but more control over the care they do receive.

For society, the trade-off is a little different: some people will be asked to do more for themselves – and will be expected to do more for themselves – so that those who need it most can get much more in the way of dedicated support.

Doctors will be expected to encourage patients to take on more responsibility for themselves, but also to have the skills to identify those who cannot. They will need to understand much better how needs vary between patients and how the needs of each patient vary over time. In the immediate aftermath of an unexpected diagnosis, most people need high levels of support and will want time when they are absolved of any expectation that they might make decisions. But equally, there are moments when people face the risk of death or disability where it might be assumed that they are unable to make judgements in their own interest, when in fact, they are both able and desperate to do so.

This is the greatest benefit of giving patients more control over their own healthcare. As individuals start to have more opportunity to determine the degree to which they are willing to take risks – whether that be risking experimental treatments to try to prolong life or risking refusing treatment to try to enjoy what remains of life

– carers and health services will become better at understanding what constitutes a good outcome and how that can be brought about.

This means that fewer people will undergo treatments that they would have refused had they properly understood what was being proposed and felt able to say no. It also means fewer people being given inadequate treatment and having their untimely end written off as something that was bound to happen. The failure to properly understand – or even recognise – the distinction between outcomes driven by patient choice and outcomes driven by medical decisions does more than anything to rob us all of our most basic rights.

The fear that patients are simply incapable or unwilling to take on this responsibility will diminish as patients live longer with illness and become more and more expert in their own diseases. The NHS will spend much more of its efforts on helping people to live with infirmity rather than curing them from illness. Attempts to firmly distinguish between what counts as "medical treatment" and what counts as "social care" will become self-evidently meaningless.

Central to this will be enabling patients to speak with more authority about their own circumstances. On one level, there is no way to dispute the indignity that is imposed by the physical limitations, discomfort, pain and lack of privacy that ill-health dictates. But the degree to which it is regarded as an indignity is in part dictated by a culture that associates good health too strongly with youth and physical integrity. In an age when more and more of the population are living with long term conditions, this will change.

These changes – and yes, once again, technology – will affect the way in which health services are arranged. More care will happen in your own home where telemedicine will reach the point of being a useful tool. More diagnostic tests and treatments will be available at local clinics. Less will happen in hospital.

For those whose life is in danger or who need complex treatment, services will be further away. Hospitals will be fewer, larger and better. The medical teams will be increasingly specialised with great depth of expertise. There will be clear and explicit standards of safety. "Never events" and medical errors will become things that really are expected never to happen. Failures in care will be monitored and will not be tolerated. The numbers of avoidable deaths – however measured – will fall.

If a time comes when further treatment is pointless, you will, if capable of it, be made aware of what is happening. You will be helped to die in comfort in your own home, if that is what you would prefer.

Rationing of healthcare will not end. But if these changes result in patients being healthier and health services more effective in their use of resources, the pressure to ration services will reduce. The extent of rationing will also depend to the degree to which, as taxpayers, we are willing to fund higher levels of care. These decisions will become easier because for the first time, we will start to properly understand where resources are improving lives and where they are making no difference – or even making things worse.

By pooling the information about our health and the care we receive, we will begin to understand which activities and which organisations are proving most successful at alleviating the burden of disease. The astonishing success that science has achieved over the last hundred years in finding new drugs and technologies to cure us will start to be applied to the way we are cared for and the way medicine is practised. Our understanding of what works in healthcare will expand beyond the laboratory and into the real world.

This will change the way that we pay for health services. We will, for the first time, be able to make sure doctors have a financial interest in making us better rather than in cutting our leg off.

By sharing our information, will each be able to see how our health, our treatment and our behaviour compares with others in similar situations. But equally, as a country, we will be able to see how our spending on healthcare is helping to improve lives.

We should not accept the assumption that, as medical technology develops, there will have to be more rationing. That need not be true if we manage our health and our healthcare resources as effectively as possible. If we make sure we only provide those treatments that fully informed patients want, we may find we have the resources to make sure that no patient is denied the treatment they need.

The aim must be to see the universal offering from the NHS start to broaden again and become more comprehensive. Most importantly, in this regard, are efforts to include social care as part of the national offer. The proposals from the Dilnott Commission are important in this regard. They have recommended that the cost of social care over a set limit be funded from national taxation replacing the current system where care is only paid for if you are unable to pay yourself. The argument against this is that only wealthier people would benefit. But one of many arguments in its favour is that it would make social care, at least in part, a universal tax funded service that we all might need to call on at some time in our lives. It would be a step towards having a true national care service.

The NHS of 1948 was based on social solidarity – the social solidarity that comes from agreeing to pool our financial resources in order to provide medical services to whoever needed them. The NHS of the future will continue to require this – but it will require more from us. In addition to paying our taxes, we will be asked to contribute two further things – time and information.

Those who are able will be expected to take on more of the work of looking after themselves. For this to happen, the main hurdle to overcome is technological. It requires information systems that make the task simple enough for people to not only be able to manage it but, more importantly, to want to do it.

That may sound overly optimistic when we look at the current state of information technology in healthcare. But the prize of getting this right is so great that it seems to me inevitable that we will get there. Technology will be slower to develop than we would like and people will adopt it at different speeds. But some things just take a bit of time.

The idea of the steam engine was around for hundreds of years – and absorbed the attention of thousands of inventors – before Thomas Newcomen and then James Watt finally cracked the problem and came up with a machine that really worked. It took over 50 years of experimentation with powered flight before the Wright brothers achieved success. Most good ideas require a great many failed attempts before the concept is honed into something that works. Innovation in information and health is no different.

Care will be needed to ensure people are not disadvantaged as these changes take place. That is where the second contribution comes in. In addition to contributing taxes and time, we will be expected provide one further element – as a nation we will be expected to pool the information we have about our lives. This needs to be done in a secure fashion that protects everyone's anonymity. But without this, it will not be possible to ensure that everyone is well cared for and that our resources have been used to best effect for all. It is through this pooling of data, more than anything, that the NHS can once again become an organisation that demonstrates how social solidarity can create healthcare that is better than anything else the world has to offer.

The NHS is sometimes accused of being too big. It is sometimes said that an organisation which employs a million people can never be sufficiently sensitive to the needs of individuals. I do not agree. I think that having a national system with the ability to introduce changes across the whole country and a common approach to the information and record-keeping is a huge advantage. More importantly, having a national organisation that encapsulates an ideal – an ideal to which the population is committed and one that we will do whatever is necessary to support – gives us the firmest foundations on which to build.

So I remain optimistic. And for one reason in particular. Why? Because we have just hosted the Olympic Games. And the Olympics are always a harbinger for this county of great things ahead.

Britain has hosted the Olympics three times. First in 1908, then in 1948 and lastly in 2012. The first two games came at crucial moments in the development of the welfare state in Britain. The 1908 games took place during the liberal reforms that established the principles of the welfare state. This was the year that Asquith took over as prime minister from Henry Campbell Bannerman and introduced the first state pensions. Shortly afterwards, in 1911, the people's budget was introduced – against fierce opposition from the Lords – and the National Insurance Act introduced compulsory health insurance for the employed. For the first time, working people were ensured access to a doctor. At that time, one in eight children died within a year of being born.

The 1948 games opened in July, the month that the NHS was founded. It was the first Olympic Games to take place in a country that guaranteed access to comprehensive modern healthcare for all its citizens regardless of ability to pay. In 1948, one in twenty deaths was caused by tuberculosis.

And the 2012 games? They come at a moment when we are re-thinking much of the way in which we look after each other as a nation. The population is more fluid – with increases in both immigration and emigration – making ties to the country more open to question. When the 1948 act was passed, healthcare was effectively made available to anyone in Britain, regardless of nationality or residency. These days, there is growing unease at the idea of foreigners coming here as health tourists. The NHS is starting to clamp down and make sure that free care is provided only to those who are legally resident. That may or may not include your neighbour.

But while we may be becoming a tad more suspicious of who should get what, our commitment to egalitarianism remains undimmed – indeed, if anything, it has sharpened. Where once access to care for all was the objective, today the objective is high quality care for all.

It seems unlikely that 2012 will go down in any history books alongside 1911 and 1948 as a pivotal moment in the history of healthcare, despite the passing of the Health and Social Care Act. But we are certainly in a period of upheaval. Within the NHS, there is the kernel of a coherent view of what the health services of the future will look like. And we are approaching a moment when we will have both the ability to change and a widespread acceptance that changes are needed.

In 1948, as the Olympics opened, the newly created NHS set the standard for what a civilised health service should look like. 2012 has seen the Olympics come and go. We are still waiting for a leap forward in our health services. But we have good reason to hope.

INDEX